Emma & I

Emma & I

The Beautiful Labrador
Who Saved My Life

Sheila Hocken

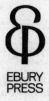

EBURY
PRESS

1 3 5 7 9 10 8 6 4 2

First published in 2011 by Ebury Press, an imprint of Ebury Publishing
A Random House Group company
First published by Victor Gollancz Ltd in 1977

The Random House Group Limited Reg. No. 954009

Addresses for companies within the Random House Group can be
found at www.randomhouse.co.uk

A CIP catalogue record for this book is available from
the British Library

The Random House Group Limited supports The Forest Stewardship Council
(FSC®), the leading international forest certification organisation. Our books
carrying the FSC label are printed on FSC® certified paper. FSC is the only
forest certification scheme endorsed by the leading environmental
organisations, including Greenpeace. Our paper procurement policy can be
found at www.randomhouse.co.uk/environment

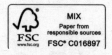

MIX
Paper from
responsible sources
FSC® C016897

Printed and bound by CPI Group (UK) Ltd, Croydon, CR0 4YY

ISBN 9780091943363

To buy books by your favourite authors and register for offers visit
www.randomhouse.co.uk

This book is dedicated to John E Coates,
ophthalmic surgeon (Mr Shearing)

Contents

1

A Child Apart

IHAD NO idea that I could not see normally until I was about seven. I lived among vague images and colours that were blurred, as if a gauze was over them. But I thought that was how everybody else saw the world. My sight gradually became worse and worse until, by my late teens, I could just about distinguish light from dark, but that was all. Even in my dreams the people had no faces. They were shapes in a fog. From my earliest recollection, waking or dreaming, the fog had always been there, and it slowly closed in until it became impenetrable and even the blurred shapes finally disappeared.

I was born in 1946 in Beeston, Nottingham. Both my parents had defective eyesight; and so did my brother Graham, who is three years older than I. The eye defect is hereditary: congenital cataracts, which in turn cause retina damage. I inherited this from my father. My mother's complaint was different, caused by German measles when she was a child, but neither parent could see much at all. The picture conjured up of the four of us – none able to see properly, yet all living together as a family – must be a strange one to a sighted person. Had I been the odd one out, a child with defective eyesight in a family where everyone could see perfectly, things would almost certainly have been otherwise. But in my family no one ever talked about blindness, or not being able to see properly. It was accepted as a fact of life, and no one mentioned it. Perhaps my mother and father kept up a sort of conspiracy of silence about it for the benefit of Graham and me, and if that was so, it was wise. What purpose could it have served to tell a boy and a girl that they were not like other children? We were spared having our confidence knocked out of us in this way.

Only in retrospect do I realise that much of what we took for granted in day-to-day life would have been considered unusual by other people. At mealtimes, knocking over a sauce bottle while feeling over the tablecloth for the salt was such a frequent happening that no one said anything when it occurred.

I must have been five or six, I suppose, before I began to think about why other children didn't run headlong into brick walls, or trip down stairs as frequently as I did. Falling down and colliding with things had always been so much a part of my life that I accepted it, and in my earliest years probably imagined myself a bit clumsy. I furnished my own explanations and excuses. At the same time, it never really bothered me.

What eventually brought home to me the fact that I was a child apart, was seeing my friends watching television. At home the whole family could not sit down to look at a programme together, because each of us had to be very close to the screen to see it at all. Suddenly I realised that other people could sit well away from the set and still see it.

My present memory of those very early days, however, is as hazy as daylight itself used to appear to me at the time. I suppose sighted people have quite a few vivid recollections of their childhood, but I can't even remember images of my mother and father then except in terms of touch and sound. And just as I don't have any visual memory of my parents, or at least, nothing that could be conveyed with any significance, I cannot remember any visual impressions of the house where we lived, which was in a little town called Sutton-in-Ashfield, near Mansfield. We moved there soon after I was born. As a home I knew it by the smell of bread baking and pies cooking, and the warmth and sound of a coal fire crackling and hissing in the grate. But no more.

My father was away a great deal, travelling round the country selling drapery at markets. No doubt his poor sight was a big handicap but he would never admit it;

the only time he would ever discuss the problem was to tell us of the funny things that happened to him.

I remember him coming home one evening after a long train journey and telling us about going into the railway cafe between trains for a cup of tea. After finding a seat in the crowds of travellers he spotted what he thought was an ashtray. He leaned forward and stubbed out his cigarette, but much to the amusement of his fellow passengers, and to his own embarrassment, the ashtray turned out to be a jam tart.

It wasn't long before my father had to admit defeat with the markets, owing to the rapid deterioration of his sight. It was a blow that completely altered our way of life. Yet children in those days did not enjoy the confidence of their parents the way they do today, and Graham and I were not told exactly what had happened. The first we knew of a change was that one day we came home from school and my mother asked us to help her start packing. She said nothing about my father's sudden failure to be able to earn a living.

'What's happening, Mum? Where are we going?' I asked.

'We've bought a shop,' she said. 'We're moving to Nottingham.'

Nottingham! This was very exciting to Graham and me – moving to the big city away from the country town where we had lived for as long as we could remember.

We did not know, as our parents did, that it was to be a step down in life, because our home was to be in one of the poorest and roughest districts of the city, St Ann's Well Road. And what neither Graham nor I realised at the time was that it would be much more difficult for us to be with new people and new children after the ones we knew and were used to.

Instead there was simply the excitement of moving. The shop was on a corner. My mother, who could see much better than my father, arranged the drapery stock, marked the prices on tickets and told my father what they were. We were used to him being on the road for long periods of time, but now he was always at home and had more time to spend with us.

Father could not help very much in the shop and – a tremendous blow to his pride – he finally had to give in to the blind way of life and make brushes at the Midland Institute for the Blind. Luckily brush-making didn't last long, for soon after starting at the Institute my father picked up a guitar for the first time. He was a natural from the very beginning, not simply strumming well known folk songs but also writing his own words and music. And now he earns his living introducing a country and western programme called *Orange Blossom Special* on Radio Nottingham. He also travels all over the British Isles playing in country and western clubs. But there is no fear of the jam tart incident recurring – he's given up smoking.

Graham and I soon found that the children in the street were rougher than the ones we had known in Sutton-in-Ashfield. They called me all kinds of names, but as my mother had always told us to, we ignored them. Probably because of this my brother and I drew closer together.

Graham was terrible at bribing me. I used to ask him to read to me when we got in bed at night. And he would say, 'I'll read you a chapter of Enid Blyton if you'll play cricket with me tomorrow.'

'Oh, no, not cricket,' I would protest. 'You know I don't like playing cricket.' I was terrified of being hit by the ball, which is very hard. In the end, though, lured by Enid Blyton and her story of 'Shadow the Sheepdog', I would relent and say, 'All right, I'll have one game of cricket with you as long as you promise not to use the hard ball.' The bargaining would then go on with Graham maintaining that it was not really cricket if you did not use a proper cricket ball, and me saying that I would not play unless he used a soft tennis ball. I usually managed to persuade him to settle for cricket with a soft ball, and he would read me my chapter.

My mother used to play with me a lot too. I had a teddy who had only one eye (ironically, it may seem) and I remember feeling permanently sorry for him. My mother and I used to play endless games with him. She took me shopping, and if we went to Woolworths I would always want to feel the toys there. I could see them as shapes, but I could attach no identity to them unless I touched them, which was possibly a problem for my mother, because the universal rule for children in those days was 'Don't touch!' But somehow she must have got the shop assistants on her side so I could feel the dolls or woolly animals or boxes of bricks. And even to this day I still do not know any object fully until I have touched it.

One incident stands out from my earliest memories. My mother took me for the day to Skegness, a popular seaside resort for people from the Nottingham area. I was on a roundabout, happily whirling in my own enclosed space, and when the ride was over I sat on my painted horse and did not get off. This was because I was accustomed to my mother coming to find me. I could never find people; instead, I always waited for them to fetch me.

So I remained on the merry-go-round. The next thing I knew, I was lifted off it by a lady with an upper-class voice. A few minutes later I was in a Lost-and-Found, terrified and howling the place down. After some time, through my tears, I made out a figure coming towards me. When the shape got close I knew it was a woman and I thought at first it was my 'rescuer'. But then, partly by her scent, I realised it was my mother. 'Oh, Mum,' I said, 'I thought you were a lady.' That phrase promptly became part of our private family language.

When I was a bit older I had a little tricycle, though I was never let out of the garden with it. But when Graham got a proper bike, I desperately wanted one as well. I plagued the life out of my parents. But, as in everything else, my mother would never say to me straight out, 'You can't have one because you can't see properly.' She would invent all sorts of excuses. It was almost as if she did not want to admit even to herself that my eyesight was not right; it was something she wished to remain buried, and never revealed. And I think my father was silent because he was disappointed that I had inherited his eye defect. I suppose that when I was born, he had hoped against hope that my eyes might be normal. But I had followed the family pattern, and I think that in a way he retreated into himself because of it, and paid less attention to me as a result. Knowing his own difficulties, he realised that things would not be any easier for me.

Yet all this simply added up to the fact, as far as I was concerned, that my brother was able to have a bike and I was not, and I didn't understand why. So, one day, I 'borrowed' my brother's shiny new Hercules. How I got on and rode it, and what followed, makes me shudder to remember even to this day. But I took the bike and wheeled it out of the gate into the road. There I rode it after a fashion without even realising that traffic kept to the left-hand side of the road. It had never struck me that cars and other vehicles kept to a specific lane. But somehow, miraculously, nothing hit me, and not knowing how to stop going down a slight hill, I turned off the road, went up the kerb and into a wall.

I had no idea what to do. The front wheel was flat, and the lamp bracket bent. My heart pounding, I left the bicycle where it lay and unsteadily found my way back home, where I hid upstairs for what seemed like hours.

Presently I heard voices from the kitchen. It was Graham, on the verge of tears, saying to my mother: 'Mum, my bike's gone. Somebody's stolen it!' Then my mother, sounding overwrought and worried: 'I haven't time to think about that. Graham, have you seen our Sheila?'

At last I summoned up courage, went downstairs and told all. I cannot remember what my mother said, but she sounded relieved to know I was safe, and did not seem to care about the bicycle. But Graham was sobbing and went out immediately to recover his bike.

Then my father came in, and my mother told him the terrible saga. He, too, was aghast rather than angry. 'Sheila,' he said, 'whatever possessed you? You might have been killed.' Then there was a silence, and I wondered what was coming next. At last he spoke. 'It's going to take your pocket money for a long time,' he said, 'to get that bike repaired ...'

It might be wondered why there were no attempts then to have my eyes operated on. The answer is that the state of eye surgery in those days was not as advanced as it is today, and my family had not been well served by the methods that were then available. My father had had a series of unsuccessful operations. My brother Graham had returned from hospital having entirely lost the use of one eye as a result of surgery (although his remaining eye was better than both of mine put together). In turn, I had had an operation; but this was not a success, and my parents, particularly with Graham's experience in mind, decided against any further attempts.

By the time I was five, the question of my education arose. I was a registered blind person and the education authorities were adamant that I should be sent away to a special school. My parents were very strongly against such a move. The attitude in schools for the blind when my father had attended one as a boy was that however much or little sight the child had, he or she had to be taught the blind way. That is, in braille. My father was not encouraged to make use of his existing sight. Things, I am very glad to say, have completely changed since then, and any child with the least bit of residual vision is encouraged to develop its use in such schools today. When my mother met my father, he could only read braille and it was she who had to teach him to read visually with the use of large print. My father, who had himself gone to a special school, had led a sheltered childhood and found it difficult later to integrate into a sighted world.

The Nottingham Education Authorities, however, had their own ideas. At first they tried persuasion, then a touch of heavy-handedness, and finally they threatened legal action if I were not 'voluntarily' sent away to a school for the blind. To this, my mother's reply was, 'Well, if I can get Sheila accepted at an ordinary primary school, then she will be receiving education, and that will be that. There'll be nothing you can do about it.' That did not go down well at all, but then we had quite a stroke of luck. It turned out that the headmaster of the local junior school that my mother approached was blind in one eye. He therefore had some understanding of the problem, but over and above that, he had compassion. He agreed to accept me, and to see how I got on. I have never stopped thanking my stars for this decision, which made such a difference to my life.

So I started at Bluebell Hill Junior School, and I remember little about it, except that it was old, noisy and overcrowded. What I do recall is how terrified I was at the swarms of children in the playground. They all seemed to be running everywhere and screaming at the same time. It was very frightening, like a sudden access to an unexpected, mad world, and at playtime I used to sit on the wall and keep out of the way, listening to the banshee noise, and at the edge of my vision seeing endless wild moving shapes. I was a small girl in a blue velvet dress who imagined herself to be one with the rest of the school, but in reality was not.

When I was eleven, I moved to Pierrepont Secondary Modern. By this time I used to go to school on my own, and the walk there was a bit like facing a 'Wall of Death' ride every day of my life. Apart from knowing I would stumble over odd objects such as milk crates left outside terrace doors, and even the steps of houses, there was also at the end of the road a crowd of boys who sometimes used to wait for me and jeer as I went by, the most complimentary of their names for me being 'Boss-eyes'. I can hear them now, 'Look at 'er … Boss-eyes …' But, strangely, these lads had a mongrel dog who took to me, and I to him. I used to pat and make a fuss of him, and sometimes he would walk to school with me. I think this was when I began to get the idea that in some cases animals are kinder than, and preferable to, human beings.

Needless to say, there were difficulties at school. The attitude was, 'Either you get on without any major additional help from us, or you really will have to be sent away to a special school.'

One of the big problems I had was not being able to see the blackboard, even if I sat in the front row. On one particular day which sticks vividly in my memory, our

English mistress, Miss Pell, gave me permission to come out and look at the board more closely. What was written was a long piece on grammar, which was very hard to take in anyway, so I had to read it a line at a time, try to remember the line, then go back to my desk to write down what I'd seen. The trouble was the class got more and more fidgety and exasperated, because every time I went out to the board I blocked off whole bits of the entire exercise that everyone else was writing straight down from their desks. Fairly soon the classroom was full of cross little requests: 'I'm doing that bit, Miss, can't you move her?' 'She's in the way, Miss.' 'Miss, she's in the light.' Miss Pell was very good. She told them, 'Well, you'll just have to wait a moment.' But the tension was building up, and after about three trips to the blackboard I gave up, and heard frustrated protests give way to sighs of relief. The silence was broken only by pens scratching while I sat back at my desk vowing I'd rather be illiterate than go through that again. The only compensation was that I was beginning to develop a very well-trained memory.

Yet for every teacher or pupil who had no consideration or proper understanding, there were as many who did, and these have very much remained in my mind. I remember a geography master who realised that I could not see the very small print and various signs and symbols on the maps and diagrams. When it dawned on him what was happening, or rather what was not happening, he offered to coach me after school. It was thoughtful and kind of him, and the dividend for us both came in the exams at the end of the year when I came second in geography.

So, given the chance, I was able to keep up with the rest, and the question never seriously arose of my having to leave and go to a school for the blind – even though my sight was becoming worse and worse. I managed to stay in the better streams, and most of my exam results were good, particularly in subjects where the teaching was to a large extent by word of mouth and I could rely on my memory. I did especially well in history and in science, where we had to do our own elementary experiments. I had little difficulty in remembering the terms of the Magna Carta, and the names of Henry's wives; nor, oddly enough, did I have any trouble manipulating a Bunsen burner. But with such subjects as geography, unless I had a teacher willing to give extra help, I was no good. At maths I was quite useless – my skill ran out on the threshold of long division. This was because I could not follow immediately the step-by-step instruction that was done with the aid of the board. The problems I had with decimal points can only be imagined.

When the time came round for the school's Parents' Day, Miss Thompson, our science teacher, decided that the pupils would dissect flowers and then place the various parts on paper, labelling them appropriately. This was something we had been doing in biology and which, because of its intricate nature, I had not been very good at. A very considerate teacher, Miss Thompson came to me and said, 'Sheila, I know you won't find it easy to do this. Would you like me to find you something else as a Parents' Day activity?'

'Yes, please,' I said immediately. I had no wish to sit on the sidelines while the other students dissected their flowers and have parents look at me and think, 'Oh, that must be the girl who can't see much.'

Unfortunately, I didn't think what Miss Thompson came up with was a very good idea. On the day of the class she said, 'I've got something for you to do, and you've got a table at the back all to yourself.' I went over to the table with her and she announced, 'There you are. There are some empty jam jars. I want you to fill them with varying amounts of water, and then you can hit them with your pencil or pen and show what different tones and noises they make.'

I was appalled. If anything would make me stand out from the rest, this would be it. 'Oh, Miss,' I said, 'can't you find me anything different to do? Couldn't I clean out the hamsters' cages?'

She appeared a little put out and replied: 'I've given this a lot of thought, Sheila. I thought it would be something you would really like to do. It's something you *can* do. You can hear it, and you can feel the water.'

'Yes, Miss, but it seems so childish, especially when everybody else is doing something really important.'

But I suppose she was very proud of the idea and she would not let me do anything else. So I had to fill the jars and hit them to make noises. All the while I could feel the eyes of the parents burning into me with pity I did not want.

I made friends at school, but not as readily as other children, mainly because I could not play the games. I used to try and join in, but could never keep up with the others. Although I was quite useless at tennis, I was always put down for it, and though I made the effort – standing there on the court in a vague sea of green dotted with moving white shapes, waving my racket around, hoping desperately that it would connect with the ball when it came over the net – I cannot remember much, if any, success. There was a striking lack of volunteers to be my partner, and I usually found myself with someone who did not like the game anyway. But I don't suppose any of this has proved a serious loss to Wimbledon!

Out of school, too, life was complicated. I had friends but, like me, they were in their teens, and at that age few are ready to respond to the needs of a blind friend who has to be looked after, and taken around. When they were going out in the evening, perhaps to the Nottingham Palais in Parliament Street, or to Jepson's, another dance hall which used to be in Hockley, I would want to go with them; but if I did go, it would mean that I had to do everything they wanted to do, and go everywhere they wanted to go. The sense of restriction was overwhelming, but there was no choice, because I would not go out on my own. When I went to dances I'd sit absolutely petrified in case a boy asked me to dance. I was so scared I would make mistakes or would not be able to follow what he was doing. On the other hand, when nobody came and asked me to dance, I was still on the edge of the chair with anxiety because, left on my own, I could not see enough, beyond a blurred sensation of light and colour and shapes moving to the music, to see where the dancers were. My constant thoughts were: 'What if they go off with their boyfriends and leave me here?' Alternating with: 'No one's asking me to dance because they can see I'm blind.' I was very mixed-up always, and confused, and often felt like a wallflower with its petals closed. I remember one particularly terrible occasion when a boy called Philip left me standing in the middle of the dance floor after the music stopped, and I could hear everyone else moving away. I felt a sense of space opening up around me as the noise of the dancers receded to the edges of the hall. I pretended to tidy my hair but inside I was panicking until one of my girlfriends came to rescue me. After that I gave up going to dances because it was such a trial. I had come to hate the whole business, and that cut me off from the rest of my age group, and meant that I had no opportunity at all to meet boys. Even when I did meet them, they tended to ignore me, and naturally I worried a lot that perhaps I would never marry.

But if life was harsher than it need have been because of my stubbornness and pride and my simple refusal to be considered apart from sighted people, there were compensations in living at home with parents who themselves knew the difficulties of blindness, and, more important, knew that the best way of dealing with them was not to give in. I was very fortunate in this. If I could not see to do something, my mother would teach me how to do it, and that was that. I would then have to get on and do it for myself. For example, the business of threading a needle. My mother taught me this by such a simple method, and one, I am sure, that a sighted person wouldn't dream of showing to someone who was blind. The method was this: take hold of the needle (the eye end can be found because it is blunter than the point) and take the piece of thread or cotton, folded double between finger and thumb. Then push the eye of the needle down between finger and thumb, and eventually the thread will go through the eye. Success is not necessarily immediate, of course. It might work first go, or it might take twenty attempts. But finally it always does succeed.

I was also taught to sew by being able to feel things. Sewing on a button, for instance, was easy, and all sorts of other mechanical actions were made possible for me by my mother teaching me how to use the sense of touch. 'Feel,' she would say. This even came down to feeling where the particles of dirt were when sweeping the floor, and feeling a second time, and a third, to make sure they had gone into the dustpan. It was the same with ironing clothes. The creases and folds can be felt. But, I suppose, had I been a blind child in a sighted family, I would never have been let near an iron for fear that I would burn myself. In my family, there was no alternative to everyone making the best of his or her lot, and that is how I was brought up.

I once asked my mother if she had had any idea before I was born that I would not have normal sight and I was appalled when she said she hadn't known one way or the other, but was willing to take the risk. Seeing my horror, she then asked me whether I'd enjoyed my life so far, and whether it had been really worth living in spite of the problems, and, of course, I had to answer that it had. She had taken a risk but I realised that she was right and that I still had the opportunity to live a full life in spite of my blindness – just as the rest of my family had.

When my last term at school came up, the decision about my future loomed large over me. What I really wanted to do was to work with dogs, because I was mad about them. At weekends I used to work at a local hoarding kennels, somehow managing to cover up the fact that I could not see properly. One Saturday, I was exercising a big Alsatian in the field, and he slipped his lead. I had no idea where he had gone and was immediately gripped by panic. What if he got out and was run over? I frantically waved his lead and collar and called and called. To my astonishment and utter relief he came back as good as gold. When I was interviewed by the careers mistress, however, and told her about wanting to work with dogs, she hardly listened. The idea was dismissed as an impossibility.

Her first question amazed me. 'Sheila, can you tell me where the North Sea is?'

North Sea? Apart from geography lessons I had been in person to Skegness, which is on the North Sea. But I could not answer. Moreover, I could not understand the reason for the question.

Next I was asked, 'Well then, where is Birmingham?'

That I knew. And the answer to the next one, 'Can you tell me where Edinburgh is?' After giving the location of Edinburgh, I summoned enough courage to ask why she wanted to know.

'Well, if you're going to be a switchboard operator,

and I'm going to recommend you, I must be sure you've got a sound knowledge of where various places are.'

I was flabbergasted. Switchboard operator! It was the last job in the world I wanted. I knew that the choice for someone with my sight was restricted, but in my wildest moments I had never thought of myself condemned to plugging and unplugging calls for a living. Even so, when term ended, I found myself on the way to the Government Training Centre at Long Eaton to have my capabilities as a switchboard operator assessed. Under the eye of an extremely brusque and strict instructor called Ted I was taught the technique of working a switchboard. Then, with the Centre's aid, I got a job with a big dress shop in Nottingham. I could still see enough at this stage to distinguish the lights on the switchboard, but I loathed every minute of it and, though it was quite easy to grasp where the various plugs went, how to hold calls, the business of taking messages and learning extension numbers, the atmosphere in the place was terrible. Yet I stuck it for a year before moving on to a rather pleasanter firm where the people were more friendly.

Coming home from work one evening I had hardly closed the front door when I heard my mother call, 'Is that you Sheila? I've got some news.'

'What's that?' I said, feeling for the peg to put my coat on.

'I've heard of a job that would just suit you.' She couldn't wait to give me all the details, and, knowing how much she worried about my going out on my own in Nottingham, I understood why she was so pleased.

The job was with a firm called Industrial Pumps. They wanted a switchboard operator. More to the point, they were not right in the middle of the city and the journey there was much easier. I rang up the following day and got through to a Mr Dickson. He didn't sound very encouraging at first, and my hopes began to fade when he said they had had so many applicants he did not really think he wanted to interview any more. But then I told him I was a registered blind person, and his attitude changed immediately.

'Why didn't you tell me that before? Come along tonight and I'll see you. Can you make half-past five?'

To my amazement I got the job on the spot, but only later did I get to know the reason why. Mr Dickson himself was disabled: one of his legs was shorter than the other and he walked with some difficulty. In fact, he turned out to be full of understanding, and not only on this occasion. He was a wonderful man, and someone who would always listen to one's problems.

As the months went by, my eyes became gradually, almost imperceptibly worse, and by the time I was seventeen I could not see where I was going, either about the house or in the street. I was now unable to read print, and had to learn braille. I came to realise how much everyday vocabulary reflects the predominance of the sighted world. Language is relatively poor in terms for precise description of sensations other than sight, and so blind people are not able to describe their perceptions very accurately. The field of reference I had become used to was shrinking. Now not only words, but ideas of time and space were inexact and arbitrary and not always in line with the notions that a sighted person would form. To those accustomed to doing it, the placing of a towel on a rail or a cup on a shelf are automatic. A blind person has to think, 'Six steps to the door, five paces down the hall to the bathroom.' Every distance has to be worked out mentally.

It was at this point – when my range of possibilities was becoming more and more limited, when my future seemed to be an ever-darkening vacuum – that Emma came into my life and totally changed it. A new world opened up for me.

2

Enter Emma

I WAS, IF the truth be known, ashamed of being blind. I refused to use a white stick, and hated asking for help. After all, I was a teenage girl, and I couldn't bear people to look at me and think I was not like them. Looking back, I must have been a terrible danger on the roads. Motorists probably had seizures; suddenly coming across me wandering vaguely through the traffic, they would have to step rapidly on their brakes. Apart from that, there were all sorts of disasters that used to strike on the way to and from work.

On the evening that made such a difference to my life, I got off the bus just about half-way home where I had to change buses, and as usual I was walking gingerly along to the right stop. Almost immediately I bumped into something. 'I'm awfully sorry,' I said and stepped forward only to collide again. When it happened a third time, I realised I had been apologising to a lamp post. This was just one of the idiotic things that constantly happened to me, and I had long since learned to put up with them or even to find them faintly amusing. So I carried on and found the bus stop, which was a request stop. No one else was there and I had to go through the scary business of trying to estimate when the bus had arrived. Generally in this situation, because I loathed showing I was blind by asking for help, I tried to guess at the sound. Sometimes I would stop a petrol tanker or a big lorry and as it drew away would stand there feeling stupid, and in the end usually managed to swallow my pride and ask someone at the stop for help.

But on this particular evening no one joined me at the stop; it was as if everyone in Nottingham had suddenly decided not to travel by bus. Of course I heard plenty of buses pass, or thought I did, but because I had given up hailing them for fear of making a fool of myself I let them all go by. I stood there alone for half an hour without stopping one, then I gave up. I decided to walk on to the next stop, hoping there would be people there.

I got along the pavement as best I could – and that is another frightening experience difficult to describe to anyone who has not been blind, because although you are surrounded by noise you have no coherent mental picture of what is around you, and are guided only by sounds. The sounds were of traffic, and people's footsteps, and sometimes I could tell by the particular quality of the sounds that I was near buildings or passing an open space. But I had absolutely no visual concept of what the road might be like, still less what might be on the other side of it – the houses, the shops, the people, and so on: this might well have been the edge of the world, or another universe for all I knew. Were there children playing, people gossiping, women buying bread or potatoes; what did they look like, who were they? I had simply no idea. I walked along in an enclosed grey little world, a box of sounds – two foot by two foot square – around me.

Eventually I reached the next bus stop. But once again there was nobody there, and no buses stopped. So I went on to the next, and then the one after that, and the one after that. By this time I was utterly lost, and simply did not know whether I was waiting at a bus stop or a telegraph post. In the end, I found myself walking about five miles back to the terminus in the city, because I knew if I got there I would be bound to catch the right bus. And this is what happened, but I was between two and three hours late getting home, and felt pretty miserable and out of sorts when I did get there.

I am a great believer in Fate. It has been the greatest single influence on my life, and I feel certain that Fate had decreed that my home teacher was there when I finally reached home that evening. Home teachers visit the blind. They come regularly to help, to talk over any problems and to supply various aids such as braille paper, braille clocks, egg timers that ring, and so on. Mr Brown, who used to visit my family (since we were all registered as blind people), was quite a feature of life while I was growing up. He was a nice man, rather like an uncle. Mother used to order wool, which could be bought more cheaply through him than at a shop. When I was young he used to bring little presents, and one of these, a doll with separate sets of clothes, I had treasured very much.

Mr Brown had been waiting for me for about an hour. I explained why I was so late, and gave all the details of my nightmare journey. He immediately asked, 'Why on earth don't you have a guide dog?'

They were the nine most important words of my life up to that time. Yet the suggestion was an astonishing one. The idea of having a guide dog had simply never occurred to me, which is strange considering my previous attachment to dogs, and my hopes of finding work with them. Perhaps it was because my sight had gone very gradually, and I had always pretended to myself that it was not really going at all, and that I could still see if I tried. I did not want to admit to being blind. In fact, I couldn't believe Mr Brown when he suggested I should apply for a guide dog. I imagined then that people had somehow to be very special to qualify for guide dogs, that only a select few had them, and, as a result I suppose, it had never crossed my mind to consider the idea at all. But Mr Brown went on, 'You quite obviously need a guide dog, and you're just the right sort of age for one.'

I really could not take the idea in. Its impact was tremendous, as if someone had taken hold of the world and completely reversed its direction. 'What do I do about applying?' I said.

He replied very firmly, and in a voice full of encouragement, 'Well, I'll tell you. I'll get you the forms, and I'll come down with them, and we'll fill them in together. I'll do the writing for you.'

When he'd gone, I sat back and thought about it. I thought of the books I had read about guide dogs. I realised it would mean I'd never again have to face the kind of terrifying business I had been through that day, blundering from bus stop to bus stop in anonymous darkness with no idea where I was. And I'd be able to go out in the evening: I could be independent!

A few days later Mr Brown was back with the forms: sheet after sheet of questions. How tall was I? What did I do for a living? What sort of house did I live in? What were my hobbies? They even wanted to know how much I weighed. We sent the forms off, and a reply came from the training centre at Leamington Spa to say that they would send a guide dog trainer to assess my personality and match me to a suitable dog. I was excited, but nervous too, because at the back of my mind I was wondering, 'What if they find I'm not suitable after all?' The prospect was heartbreaking. When the trainer came, he went along with me to see where I worked and what I did. We went for a walk together so that he could test my walking pace, and see I had no odd characteristics, such as skips and hops, and so on when I went round corners. He examined the house we lived in, which had virtually no back garden and no fencing, and said, when I explained we were hoping to move to a council house, 'You must have a garden well fenced-off for your dog.' Lastly, he told me that there was a waiting list for guide dogs, and it would be about nine months to a year before I finally had a dog of my own.

This was in November 1965. The waiting period was an agony of frustration. Every time a letter came I seized it, and tried to find someone to read it to me as quickly as possible. During these months I had plenty of time to find out about the Guide Dog Association. It was started in 1934, but the original idea of using dogs to lead blind people was born in Germany during the 1914–18 war, when a doctor, in charge of some men blinded at the front, one day left his Alsatian to look after a soldier, and was struck by the way the dog carried out his task. The idea spread across the Atlantic and back to England. Yet, unbelievably, the use of guide dogs was opposed here at first because people thought it unnatural, cruel even, for dogs to be put to work in this way. Fortunately, the Association flourished through a lot of hard work and voluntary effort. Today there are four centres for training guide dogs and their owners, at Bolton, Exeter, Forfar and Leamington Spa, as well as headquarters at Ealing near London, and a Breeding and Puppy-Walking Centre near Warwick.

I also learned that some blind applicants had to be rejected for various reasons, and this worried me. But the letter I wanted so much came more quickly than I had thought possible. It arrived towards the end of the following May, and I had only five more weeks to wait. Would I be at the training centre, Leamington Spa, on 1 July? Would I? I was prepared to camp on their doorstep so as not to miss the day.

At last, 1 July arrived. It was, as I thought only proper, glorious weather – bright and sunny. Obviously I could not have got from Nottingham to Leamington Spa on my own. But I was very lucky. Geoff, one of the reps at the firm where I worked, had offered to take me in his car. I was up with my cases packed and ready long before he called for me at nine o'clock. We took the M1 south from Nottingham, Geoff doing his best to describe the scenery to me as we went. I disliked travel-ling, as there was nothing to occupy me except the business of going from A to B. Geoff's descriptions at least stopped the boredom. Yet I couldn't really imagine all the things he was telling me about. I had no mental picture of what fields looked like because I couldn't remember ever seeing one, much less a cow. I remember him saying to me, 'What do you think I look like? You must have an *idea* of what I look like.'

'Yes, I get an image when I hear people, just as you must get an image of what people look like in your imagination when you hear them on the radio. But,' I added, 'if you later see a photograph of what they're really like, the two images don't match up, do they?'

'No, you're right. They don't,' he said.

'Well, don't blame me if I've got the wrong idea of you ... I think you've got dark, curly hair, and I know that you're about five foot seven because I can judge that when you're standing up and you talk.'

'Mm,' he replied, non-committally. Then he went on, 'Do you ever feel people's faces to get an image of them?' I told him I didn't, but not the reason. It would have been like telling everyone I couldn't see.

About halfway to Leamington, Geoff asked if I'd like to stop for coffee. I did not really want to. For one thing I wanted to get to Leamington as quickly as possible. For another, I hated going into strange places where I knew there would be lots of people, because I always felt so embarrassed. But we did stop, mainly because I thought Geoff deserved a coffee. We drew off the motorway, and into a big car park. Geoff wanted to be helpful, and he grasped my arm, not realising how unnerving it was for me being dragged along in this way. As he was taking me from the car park, he said, 'Steps here, Sheila.' That was fine, as far as it went. But he didn't say whether the steps went up or down. I assumed they went up. I was wrong. I suppose I ought to have asked, to make sure. Then he led me, or more accurately propelled me, through some doors. I got the impression we were in a very large room, full of women, all talking. I could smell their perfume, and the coffee. I imagined it was about eleven o'clock, and they were all in there for the coffee break.

Left alone while Geoff got the coffee, I panicked. I felt desperately cut off, and wanted to run. Then another embarrassment presented itself. I wanted to go to the toilet. But I did not want to have to ask Geoff. Although the situation was not new to me, I always found it humiliating. Unfailingly, it took me right back to primary school, my hand sawing the air, 'Please teacher, can I leave the room?' When I did summon up the courage to mention my predicament Geoff was very good and said immediately, 'Oh, of course. I'll get someone to take you.' Either he didn't notice my embarrassment, or covered up very well. He left the table and went to speak to someone. As it turned out, he must have picked the biggest and strongest woman in the room. I had the bruises on my arm the next day to prove it. She got hold of me and hauled me out of my seat by brute force. 'Come along, my dear,' she boomed, 'I'll take you. You poor thing, not being able to see.' And she literally pushed me through the room. I crashed into everything possible on the way: tables, chairs, even an occasional cup and saucer, they all went flying. I felt like a red-faced bull in a china shop. Even when I was in the Ladies, she insisted on standing guard outside the door, enquiring from time to time, 'Are you all right, dear?' and 'You're sure you don't need any help?' I didn't know whether to laugh or cry. I could not wait, once released from the grip of this Amazon, to be back in the car and driving the last lap to Leamington.

The training centre, Geoff told me when we arrived, was a large, Tudor-style house, with trees all round it, standing in a great expanse of grounds. While we waited for someone to come and look after me, I had a sudden moment of misgiving. 'What,' I thought, 'if I go through the course, and I can't do whatever they teach, and they say I'm not good enough to have a guide dog. What then?' It was a cold, alien feeling and I was shaking slightly when the receptionist arrived.

She instantly dispelled my momentary panic. 'Hello, Sheila, we were expecting you round about this time. If you'd like to take my arm, I'll show you to your room.' No pushing or dragging here, I thought. Geoff said goodbye, and the receptionist took me through a lot of corridors and up several staircases. It seemed an enormous place as she guided me along, explaining the layout of the centre, and the way to the dining-room, the lounge, the bathroom and toilets, and so on. Then we reached my room. 'Here we are,' said the receptionist, 'Number Ten.' She stopped and told me to put my hand up to the door. To my utter amazement I felt 'Number Ten' in braille. 'All the doors are numbered or marked like this,' she said, 'so you won't have any trouble finding your way about.' I was quite staggered. At last a place where they really understood the business of being blind. I felt better just at the touch of the 'Number Ten' on my door. Imagine, I thought, as I felt the outline through my fingers, they actually *expect* you to feel your way about.

Then the receptionist took me into my room, and described the layout. I, of course, had to 'picture' it through my sense of touch and my estimation of the distance between obstacles. Directly behind the door was an easy chair and then a fitted wardrobe. I felt along the wall and found my bed, and along the bed to the radio and the table. In the corner was a handbasin with hot and cold taps, and on the same wall was the dressing table. I discovered a looking glass on the dressing table, and the receptionist must have noticed my expression. 'Ah yes,' I heard her say, 'the looking glass. You want to know why. Well, the reason is that if we didn't have normal fittings such as mirrors and lamps in the rooms it would be very odd to the sighted, particularly to those who work here. We expect you to fit into a sighted world, and accept these sorts of things.' Wonderful, I thought – integration ...

There was just one more item of furniture left to examine, and it was the most important. Next to the dressing table was the dog bed. It seemed massive, and I felt its interior-sprung mattress and blanket. It was so obviously comfortable I fancied it myself. When I'd finished identifying it by touch the receptionist said, 'Well that's it, Sheila. I'll leave you to unpack. The midday meal will be in half an hour.' I heard the door close behind her, and started unpacking my suitcases. On the way to the wardrobe I had to keep passing the dog bed. Every time I did so I stopped and felt it. I wondered longingly what sort of dog would soon be sleeping in it.

The sound of knocking interrupted my thoughts. When I opened the door, a voice said, 'Hello, I'm Brian Peel. I'm your trainer.' He not only trained the dogs, but also taught people how to use them. His handshake felt firm and friendly; I was sure we would get on well. 'If you'd like to come down with me,' he went on, 'I'll show you exactly where the dining room and lounge are.' We went down to the lounge, and he explained the geography of the room. 'We meet here each morning to begin the day's training. There are chairs round the outside. If you follow them round to the right, you'll find the radio and television. On the opposite side are braille books and games ... mind that coffee table ... if you remember that table stands where the carpet ends, you won't walk into it.'

As we went on to the dining room, the prospect of a familiar ordeal loomed up in my mind. I hated eating meals with sighted people. It always led to some kind of embarrassment. They usually wanted to cut my meat up, and imagined it would be better if I ate with a spoon instead of with a knife and fork. Or they said, 'Oh dear, if only I'd known you couldn't see, I would have made sandwiches.' I would become so demoralised and nervous I could hardly eat at all when a plate of food was eventually put in front of me. Not knowing what was on it, much less exactly where the food was, I would stab away, usually missing potatoes or meat or whatever, and ending up bringing my teeth together on the metal of an empty fork.

At the training centre it was totally different. Brian sat next to me and put the plate in front of me. 'Here we are,' he said, 'Fish, chips and peas. Chips at twelve o'clock, peas at three o'clock and fish between nine and six.' So I not only knew what I was going to eat, but where to find it. We talked during the meal. 'Are there any other people here for training?' I asked.

'You're the first to arrive,' said Brian, 'we've three more coming this afternoon.'

Then, before many more chips and peas had disappeared, I asked the question which was burning in my mind: 'When do we get our dogs?'

'In a day or two, when we know a little bit more about you and you know more about the dogs. You know, a lot of the people we get for training have never had even a pet dog before they come here, and they wouldn't know how to look after a guide dog. So first we teach the business of actually looking after a dog. Then, of course, you can't work with a dog unless you know how she's been trained, and what commands she will respond to.'

'I see,' I said. There was a pause. Then I asked, 'Have you chosen the dog I'm going to have?'

'I think so,' said Brian, 'but over the next two days I shall make absolutely sure. You see, I know the dogs, but I don't know the students properly yet, even though you've all filled in your questionnaires. The thing is, we match the dog to the future owner as far as possible. For instance, if an owner is young and can move quickly, we want a dog that can move quickly. If the owner's older, we want a dog that will slow down a bit, and, generally, we try to match characteristics. Your dog – or the one I *think* you're going to have – was puppy-walked by a woman who had no men living in the house; she's obviously a woman's dog – she gets on with them better than with men. She's quite sensitive, too, and because you've handled dogs before, we think you might suit one another. But even so, like everyone on the course, you'll have to get used to her.'

After the meal, we went back to the lounge, and met the other students who had arrived in the meantime. Two of them I got to know very well. There was Dotty (Dorothy, officially), who was about thirty-four. She had come for her second guide dog. And there was Harry, a man of forty-nine who had been blinded during the war. He had come for his third guide dog.

During the afternoon, Brian began to tell us what to expect in the month ahead. He told us how he trained the dogs, and how we would be trained to use them. With two people present who had already had guide dogs, I felt a very raw recruit, and slightly uneasy. But I need not have. Brian explained that even for people who had had a guide dog before, it was necessary to come back to the centre, and retrain with their new dog. Techniques of handling were constantly being improved, and a dog had to have a month with its new owner to transfer its allegiance and affection away from the trainer.

In the evening, Dotty and Harry told me about their previous dogs, and it was exciting to hear about them. But when the time came to go to bed, and I went upstairs to my room, I felt very lonely. In the room next to mine, I heard Dorothy's radio and decided to knock on her door.

'It's Sheila, may I come in?'

'Of course, the chair's behind the door. Sit down.'

I sat down and tried to make conversation, but Dotty didn't seem very communicative. In fact, she sounded rather upset.

'Would you rather I went?'

'Oh no, please don't.'

So I tried to cheer her up. 'Aren't you looking forward to getting your new dog? I can't wait to get mine.' At this, to my amazement, she burst into tears. 'Oh dear,' I said, 'whatever's the matter? What have I said?'

'It's all right,' she sobbed, 'I shall be all right. But I don't want another dog.'

I was utterly at a loss. 'Don't want another dog? I don't understand.'

'Well,' she said, 'you'd understand if you'd left a dog behind.' And it emerged that Paddy, her old dog, had had to be retired early because of illness, and had gone to friends near Dotty's home. 'It's so *awful*,' she went on, 'to have left Paddy behind, and to come for another dog. I feel I've betrayed her.'

I tried to console her. 'But if Paddy couldn't go on working, I'm sure she'll be glad to see another dog in her place ...'

'I don't know …'

'But *surely,* for your own sake you must try to transfer your affection.'

'Yes. I know you're right. But it's easier said than done. At the moment I just don't feel able to love another dog.'

There was nothing more I could do to help. I said 'Goodnight' in as kindly a way as I could.

Next morning, all the gloom was swept away. At about half-past seven I was woken by a great chorus, not far away, of barking dogs. It was the sweetest music I had heard for years. Which one, I wondered lying there half-awake, is going to be mine? Which bark is hers? I hurried through breakfast. I wanted to get down to the instruction as soon as possible. When we had all assembled in the lounge, we were each issued with a white harness for our dogs, and, so we would get the hang of using it, there was a life-size plastic model of a guide dog. We called him Fred.

'Your dogs,' Brian began, 'are used to working with experienced sighted trainers. They won't take kindly to you blundering round them like blind people, trying to find out where to put the harness on. This is where Fred comes in. You can practise on him first.'

After we had all, in turn, found the correct end of Fred, Brian continued to instruct us on how to position ourselves by the dog: the dog always being on the left.

'These exercises,' Brian went on, 'may seem trivial. But you will be getting a fully trained dog. The least you can do is to try to give the impression that you are a fully trained owner.'

Positioned at Fred's side, I was told how to instruct him. 'Let's pretend you are telling your dog to go forward. Always indicate with your right arm which direction you want. This will help the dog.' My first effort was unbelievably feeble. Brian started laughing. 'Well, if you were going to start off in the direction you were pointing you'd be leaping over your dog's head. Now have another go. No. Don't stand behind him, you'll step on his tail.' And so on. It was as well we had Fred to practise on. At least his plastic tail was not sensitive to my foot.

Our next lesson was to learn how to follow the dog. Brian played the part of the dog, because Fred had not yet been fixed up with wheels. With dummy harness, and Brian in the lead, we set out in the grounds of the training centre. It was very difficult to follow, and to stop and go when he did. I was sure I had two left feet, and by the end of the first day's training I was convinced I would never make a guide dog owner. But I was determined to improve and already the feel of the harness had come to be important to me.

In the lounge after breakfast the following day there was tremendous expectancy and excitement because we all knew we were going to meet our dogs for the first time. Brian gave us a final briefing, and then asked us to go back to our rooms. 'There'll be less distraction there,' he said, 'and you'll get to know your dog, and vice versa, with a bit of peace and quiet.'

I went up to Number Ten – able to find my way now unaided. I sat on the edge of the bed waiting, with the door open, and with enough time to have a stray, disturbing thought: 'What if my dog doesn't like me? What if she stands growling at me?' Then I heard Brian's footsteps approaching along the corridor, and with them I heard the clicking patter of a dog's paws.

'Here we are, Sheila,' said Brian as he came into the room, 'here's your dog. She's called Emma, and she's a chocolate-coloured Labrador.'

At the same time I heard a tail swishing the air, and Brian leaving, closing the door behind him. 'Emma,' I called. Immediately she came bounding across the room, and suddenly I was nearly bowled off the bed. Then I was licked all over. 'Hello, Emma,' I said, 'hello.' I could hardly believe it. She kept licking me, and pushing her cold nose into my hands. I knew then we were going to get on together. She likes me, I thought. She *likes* me. I could have danced round the room.

I tried to feel the shape of her head, but she would not stop bouncing up and down in front of me, twisting, turning and making snuffling noises in my hands. Every now and then I got a wet nose in my face. But at last she settled and sat by my feet, and I was able to feel what she was like. Her coat was very thick and rough, reminding me of a teddy bear's. She was smallish for a Labrador, not fat, but thickset. She had a very thick tail, and ears that were as soft as velvet. And she was so lively.

Emma did not give me long to run my hands over her. She started to fetch me things. Under the dressing table I kept my shoes. She began rushing after them, and bringing them to me one by one. The message was quite clear. 'Here I am. I'm Emma. I'm your new dog, and this is your gift, a shoe.' I could not remember ever being so happy before. And from those first few moments of greeting, Emma's affection has never wavered. From then on she was never to leave my side, and I, in turn, took on the responsibility for her every need.

3

Training

M Y FIRST WALK with Emma came that afternoon, and it was immediately evident why we had to have a month's training with the dogs. Although Emma took to me, and we got on well together, she would not do a thing I told her. She would obey no one but Brian. Attachment and obedience to me would clearly come only with training.

I put Emma's harness on, and we started off down a quiet road near the centre. Brian was standing next to us. He gave the command to go forward, but before he even got the '-ward' bit out we were off, several miles down the road it seemed, and I was galloping along, hanging on grimly to the harness.

'I'll never keep this up,' I managed to gasp.

'Oh, you'll soon get used to it,' said Brian. 'You'll get fitter as you go along. The trouble is you've been accustomed to walking so slowly.'

A guide dog's pace apparently averages about four

miles an hour. This compares with an ordinary sighted person's two to three miles an hour. So what kind of speed I used to achieve before, I have no idea, but it was obviously not competitive even with that of the snail population. At last I began to settle down to the fast rhythm, and was just beginning to think I might enjoy it after all, when, without any warning whatsoever, Emma stopped. I was off the pavement before I could pull up. Emma had sat down on the kerb, and I heard Brian laughing.

'Don't go without your dog, that's Lesson Number One,' Brian said. 'If you go sailing on when she stops at the kerb, you'll get run over. She stops, you stop.'

'Well, I didn't know she was going to stop, did I? And you didn't tell me.'

'No, you're right. But you've got to learn to follow your dog.'

Brian was about twenty-eight at the time, very pleasant and with a great sense of humour. I imagined him good-looking with fair hair and glasses. I liked him especially because he refused to make concessions to our blindness. He expected us to be independent. Rather than mop us up, and say, 'There, there,' when we fell off the kerb, he would turn it into a joke, which was the best medicine. At least it was for me. It certainly made me get up and think, 'Right. I'll show you who can be a good guide dog owner.'

So on this occasion I got back behind Emma, took up the harness again, and said, 'What next?'

'You've got to cross this road. First you listen for any traffic. If it's quiet, you give Emma the command to go forward.'

When I could hear no traffic, this is what I did. But nothing happened.

Brian said, 'She knows that you're behind her and not me. You've got to encourage her, to make her want to take you over the road.'

'Good girl, Emma,' I said, 'there's a clever dog.' And after a little more of this persuasion, and the word 'Forward', thrown in from time to time, she finally took me across the road.

Crossing the road with a guide dog is a matter of teamwork: whatever you do, you do it together. I have met sighted people with such weird ideas about this. Either they think the dogs are not very clever, but just wear the harness to show their owner is blind – a sort of plea for help – or they think the dogs are super-human, and the blind people idiots who are being taken round for a walk rather as other people take their dogs. The importance of partnership, or even its existence, never seems to occur to most people. My job when crossing a road was to listen and Emma's was to look. Only when I could hear nothing should I give her the command to cross. But if I was wrong in my assessment of the traffic, and she could see something coming, she would wait until it was clear.

Guide dogs are taught to stop and sit down at every kerb and wait for the next command. The four basic commands are, 'Right', 'Left', 'Back' and 'Forward'. And you have to position yourself with your dog so that you give her every opportunity to obey the right command. For instance, when the command to go forward is given, it is accompanied by an indication in that direction with the arm. It is also important to keep talking to the dog, and Brian reminded me of this on our first walk, just after we had crossed the road.

'Don't stop talking, or Emma'll think you've fallen asleep.'

'What do I say?' I asked rather stupidly.

'It doesn't matter, as long as you make it interesting. Tell her what you had for breakfast if you like.'

So there I was, galloping along a street in Leamington discussing bacon and eggs with a chocolate-coloured Labrador. Brian went on, 'You're working together, and if you stop talking, she'll stop working. You've got to keep her interest. She's a dog, and there are lots of nice, interesting smells all round, and things passing that you can't see. So unless you talk to her, she'll get distracted and stop to sniff a lamp post.' I was quite hoarse by the time we had finished our first walk together.

I owe a great deal to Brian, not only for his training,

but also for matching Emma and me together. His assessment of all he knew about us resulted in an inspired pairing, as time was to prove.

One day I remember asking him where Emma came from. What I really meant was, how did the centres come by the guide dogs? Brian explained that they came to Leamington, or one of the other centres, after being puppy-walked. The Guide Dog Association has a big breeding and puppy-walking centre at Tollgate House, near Warwick. They own a number of brood bitches and stud dogs that are let out to people as pets, because, naturally, a permanent kennel life is not desirable, and living with a family is a much happier arrangement. At the same time the Association controls which dog should mate with which. When the litters come along, it picks the dogs or bitches required for training. At about eight weeks old, a puppy undergoes various tests to see if it is basically bold and friendly, and capable of being trained as a guide dog. Dogs bred in this way form about sixty per cent of the total, and there are now about two thousand guide dog owners in the country. The remaining forty per cent come to the Association either by purchase or donation from breeders or private individuals. But the rejection rate is high. Dogs are kept on approval for about three weeks to see if they are suitable. If they're not, they're returned to their owners. In all cases the dogs chosen are usually female, because the male dog has a rather different outlook and nature, including a territorial instinct, and is not as tractable as the female, who in any case is spayed for the purposes of being a guide dog. About seventy per cent of the breeds used are Labradors, like Emma – though I prefer to think she is unique, even among Labradors – and the remainder Alsatians, Collies, Golden Retrievers, and crosses from all of these.

Once the selection is made, the puppies go to people called puppy-walkers, who live around the training centres, and give homes to potential guide dogs for about a year. In this time they have to teach the dog the basics. The dogs learn how to be well-mannered and clean in the house, to keep off furniture, not to beg for food and to obey commands such as 'Sit', 'Stay', 'Down', 'Come', and so on. They are taught to walk on a lead, but not at heel, because of course they will eventually be required to walk in front of a blind man or woman. In general, the puppy-walkers are expected to take the dog everywhere with them, so that the dog is not shy of traffic, buses or trains, or the sort of sudden noises that sometimes occur in the street, such as pneumatic drills. They are also specifically instructed to take the dogs shopping. During this phase the puppy grows up and becomes used to urban life, and at the same time should remain bold and friendly.

At this point, Brian told me, they come to the centres

for guiding training, which lasts about five months. The puppy-walkers do a wonderful job. I couldn't do it myself: have a dog for a year, then part with it; then have another, and see it go, and so on, and I really admire those who do so much to forge the first essential link between dog and blind person.

Naturally, when Brian told me all this, I wanted to know who had puppy-walked Emma, and he said, 'Someone called Paddy Wansborough. She's a marvellous woman. She's given nine or ten dogs to the Association after puppy-walking them. In fact, Emma wasn't bred by the Association. She was given to Paddy as a puppy, given her basic year, and then donated to the Association.'

I determined that one of the first things I would do when I got home would be to contact Paddy Wansborough.

Next day, I was out with Emma again. As the training progressed I gradually got more used to her. We used a minibus to get us about Leamington, and this played a big part in the training, because it taught us how to use public transport. When we were on the bus and the dogs under the seats, I heard a great bellow from Brian, 'I can see two brown paws sticking out.' Brown paws, I thought, that must be Emma.

He went on, 'Do you want somebody to stand on her?'

'No, of course I don't.'

'Well, do something about it.'

I began to wonder if my first impressions of Brian had been wrong. But though he was shouting at me a lot, he must have guessed what I was thinking.

'No one else is going to tell you these things, Sheila. If you don't learn here, Emma'll be the one that suffers, not you.'

My trust in Emma grew daily, but I really knew she had transferred her affections from Brian to me on about the tenth day of my stay at the centre. Up to then, she had always slept until morning in her dog bed on the other side of the room. But on this particular evening, she refused to go to her bed. Instead, she curled up on the floor as near to my pillow as she could get. I felt then that we had made it. We were a team, each needing the other's company. I woke the following morning with an odd sensation. It felt as if there were a steamroller on my chest. Emma was sitting on top of me, pushing with her nose, telling me, I have no doubt at all, that it was time for us both to get up. She was full of life and exuberance, and could not wait to start the day. When I did get up, I could hear her shake herself in anticipation, and stand wagging her tail near the door.

One of the centre's ingenious ways of familiarising us with the day's programme was by using tactile maps. Pavements, buildings, and so on were raised on a wooden map of Leamington, so we could feel our way over the routes beforehand, right down to the zebra crossings and the bus stops. Emma would find these things for me, but I had to be in the right road, and the map helped enormously to make sure we did not miss our way. Our walks became more and more complicated, and Brian would try to find places where there were road works, to ensure we had mastered the business of getting round them, as well as other obstacles. Bus trips and shopping expeditions were also in the curriculum, and I really enjoyed shopping with Emma. She would not only find the shop, but also take me up to the counter. I began to forget I was blind. No one fussed round me any longer. They were all too interested in Emma.

But things did not always go smoothly. I was not keen on the obstacle course we had to practise. Emma always reacted very quickly, and usually I was not fast enough to follow. She would see the obstacle, assess it, and take a snap decision which way to go. Before I knew what was happening she would have changed course to one side or the other, and I would be left in a trail of harness and confusion. Brian always seemed to be on hand when I made mistakes, even if I thought he was following some other student. I would suddenly hear a great shout: 'When your dog jumps, you jump.'

It was easier said than done. On occasions like this,

Emma would lose confidence and sit down immediately. It was almost as if she were saying, 'It's no good me doing my bit, if all you can do is to trail behind and finish up in a heap.' The only way I could get her back to work again was to apologise and promise to do better next time.

It was while we were doing the obstacle course that I learned one of Emma's aversions. It came to our turn and we were going through the obstacles fairly well. All at once Emma shot off like a rocket, and I felt myself being taken at right angles up a steep grass bank. As we went, I heard Brian hysterical with laughter. When we finally came to a stop, I said rather breathlessly, 'What was all that about? Whatever did she do that for?'

'Oh, it's Napoleon.'

'Napoleon? What do you mean, Napoleon?' I thought Brian had suddenly gone out of his mind.

'You know,' he said, 'the cat. Napoleon, the cat.'

'Oh,' I said. But I still did not know why Emma had shot up the bank.

Brian, still laughing, explained that Emma could not stand cats. She knew better than to chase them, but if she saw one, she would take off in the opposite direction – the opposite direction in this case having been the steep grassy bank. Still, Brian did congratulate me on my alacrity and speed in following, and promised to keep us in mind if there was ever a guide dog expedition to Everest. At the same time, I thought that the only way to cure Emma of her dislike of cats would be to get one, and I put that on my list of resolutions for when I got home.

That evening as we were sitting in the lounge, Brian came in and we laughed again about Emma and the cat. Then I asked him something that fascinated me more and more the longer the course went on. How did they train the dogs to accomplish the amazing things they did for us? I knew a little about dog training from the experience I had had with them, but I could not fathom some of the dogs' abilities. After all, it is a fairly simple matter to train a dog to sit at a kerb every time, but how do you train them to disobey you? I asked Brian, 'For instance, I told Emma to go forward yesterday, when I hadn't heard a car coming, and she wouldn't go because she'd seen one. How on earth do you train them to do that?'

Brian replied, 'Once you've got a dog basically trained, and you're waiting to cross the road, you see a car coming and tell the dog to go forward. The dog, naturally, obeys immediately, but you don't move, and the car – other trainers drive them for these exercises – hoots, and makes a lot of noise, and the dog comes back on the pavement; by repetition of this sort of thing the dog is conditioned to associate the moving vehicle with danger, and therefore, despite all instinct to obey, refuses to move even when the command is given. Of course, only fairly intelligent dogs will respond like this, and that's why we have to be very stringent with our tests of character and aptitude to begin with.'

'What about obstacles?' I asked.

Brian explained that the principle behind teaching dogs not to walk their owners into obstacles was to get the dog to associate an obstacle with displeasure – to use a mild word – and also distress. A start is made with something simple such as a post. The dog walks the trainer into the post, is immediately stopped, the post is banged to draw attention to it, and the right way, allowing room, is shown. The next time a forceful 'NO' is shouted when the post is collided with, and the right way is shown again. So by repetition the dog eventually gets the message, and at the same time, the range of obstacles is extended to include the most frequent pavement obstacles of all, people.

It sounded simple in a way, but I knew a lot of hard work and talented training went into all this. The trainers, Brian told me, worked with a blindfold on when they considered the dogs had reached a certain standard of proficiency. They did this for about a fortnight to create real working conditions for the dogs, and give them confidence through working with someone they knew.

It was interesting to hear Brian explain it all, and particularly, in the light of what followed in the last stage of the course, the disobedience part. We were nearing the end of our month at Leamington, and went out once more in the minibus. Emma's paws, by now, were always well tucked away. Brian told us we were going to the railway station as a final test.

I have always loathed railway stations because of the noise, the hundred and one different obstacles, and the general sense of bustle which, if you are blind, is scary. I got to dislike them so much I would never go into one, still less travel by train, even if there were a sighted person to take me. But Brian was adamant. 'Well, you know, you've got to get used to it. You might want to go by rail one day, or meet somebody off a train, and you've got Emma to guide you now. She knows her way around. There's nothing to it.'

I was not convinced. We got to the station, and I put Emma's harness on. Brian said, 'Right. I'll just go and park. You go in; Emma knows the way. I'll be with you in a minute or two.'

Emma took me through the doors, down a couple of flights of steps, in and out between people on the platform and sat down. I had no idea where I was. I just stood and waited for Brian. He was there within a couple of minutes. 'Right,' he said, 'Emma's sitting bang on the edge of the platform. There's about a six-foot drop in front of you to the railway line. Now tell her to go forward.'

I was petrified, and could feel my spine tingle. 'You must be joking,' I said.

'No, go on. Tell her to go forward.'

I stood there, not knowing what to do. This really was a terrible test. Dare I do it? I was so scared, I felt sick. In that moment I really did not want a guide dog. Everything I had heard about them, all the training we had done, all I felt about Emma flashed through my mind, and it meant nothing. I just wanted, there and then, to lay the harness handle on Emma's back and leave, get out, escape, anything. But, in a sort of hoarse whisper, I heard myself saying, 'Forward.'

Immediately, up she got, and almost in the same motion pushed herself in front of my legs. Then she started pushing me back, right away from the edge of the platform.

I have never felt so ashamed in all my life. I felt about an inch tall. How could I possibly have been so doubting, so unworthy of Emma? I was utterly humiliated. Brian said, 'There you are. I told you Emma would look after you, whatever you do. Whatever you tell her to do, if there's any danger in front of you, she'll push you away.'

So that was it. We had made it. The sense of freedom was incredible. I got over my awful feelings of shame, because I sensed that Emma understood and forgave. That afternoon I walked with her down the Parade in

Leamington, the busy main road, crowded with shoppers. I walked with a great big smile on my face, weaving in and out of all those people, and feeling: I don't care if you can *see* I'm blind. I can see too: I've got Emma, and she's all I need.

4

Home Again

ALL TOO SOON the day came when we were to go home, Emma and I. It was, oddly enough, very sad. It happened to be raining – pouring down – and the weather matched my mood. Even though I could not see the rain, I felt very grey and depressed. I hated the idea of having to leave the centre and all the friends I had made. Even more, I really did not want to go home, although I now had Emma, and kept trying to convince myself that things back in Nottingham were *bound* to be different. I was afraid that somehow I might be enveloped in the old ways again, despite Emma. I had not yet grasped to what an enormous extent she was about to change my life. I still had to learn to put my confidence in her.

Heavy with misgivings, I left Leamington with Emma on her harness beside me. The two of us arrived in Nottingham, were met and taken home. Once home, I let Emma off the lead and took off her harness: she went wild. Everyone was immediately taken with her. She bounded all over the place, through every room, round and round; I could hear her tearing about, sending rugs flying, stopping to sniff each chair and table leg. The air swished to the wagging of her tail, and resounded with her snortings and sniffings. This, she obviously realised, was where she was going to live. It was such a different Emma from the sober responsible animal on the harness, and for the first time I appreciated that there were two distinct sides to her character: one when she was working, and in charge of me, and the other when she was off the harness, totally joyous, full of fun and energy, and as far from any sense of responsibility as a clown. My misgivings began to evaporate.

That first night back, Emma slept at the bottom of the bed; she had decided that there was no other place good enough for her, and in the morning she woke me with her usual insistence. It struck me that this morning we were really starting a new life together. We would be going out into Nottingham on our own. I got out of bed and started dressing. This was not my usual form, because I'm normally a very slow, sleepy starter, but on this day of all days I could not wait to find out how Emma and I, put to the test, would get on together.

Over breakfast I decided we would go to visit some old friends, Norman and Yvonne, whom I hadn't seen recently and who lived quite near. In the decision itself lay the prospect of freedom. With Emma, I would be able to go all over Nottingham!

I had the directions worked out in my mind after a telephone consultation. They presented no problems: all I had to do was to go out of our front gate, tell Emma to turn right to the top of the road, a main road, turn right again, go straight to the bottom, turn left, and ask her to find the first gate. So, off we went.

Twenty minutes after setting out, we were standing in the porch of Norman and Yvonne's house, and I was feeling for the bell. We had done it. To anyone walking down that Nottingham street of detached houses, lined with trees and built in the 1920s, there may have appeared nothing out of the ordinary about a girl and a dog standing in a doorway waiting for the bell to be answered. But inside me was a huge sense of triumph: it was a milestone. 'Good girl, Emma,' I kept saying. I was so proud of her.

Norman and Yvonne were naturally delighted to see me, and they were even more thrilled to meet Emma. They made a great fuss of her. Several hours later we set off home, and found our way back to the main road. Then came a terrible realisation. In my excitement that everything was going so well with Emma, I had forgotten to count how many intersections we had crossed. There had been no need to count on the way there because we went as far as the road went, up to a T-junction. But I should have counted for getting back. And I hadn't. So there I was with no idea where I should tell Emma to turn left. After a whole month of training, I had straightaway forgotten one of the cardinal principles: always count the roads as you go.

What could I do? I thought: 'Here I am, and there's no trainer to save me.' Emma, all unknowing, was taking me along at her furious pace, and I felt as if I were in an endless race to nowhere. Not only that, but I felt I had let Emma down. I seemed alienated from her through my own eagerness and thoughtlessness; I was sure, too, that she would never commit a mistake that would put us both in jeopardy. Emma wasn't in the least daunted, however, and, ignoring my commands, started taking me down a side road. I tried to stop her. 'No, Emma. No! Go back, go back!' But she paid no attention. In turn, I dared not let go of her, so I had to follow. At last she turned left again, and sat down. Instinctively I put my hand out. I felt leaded-lights and painted wood with one or two blisters. It was my back door. If I had forgotten to count the roads on the way out, Emma certainly hadn't!

Not long after we were home from Leamington I wrote to Paddy Wansborough, the marvellous woman who had puppy-walked Emma. By 'wrote' I mean, technically speaking, that I sent a tape-recorded cassette to tell her how much Emma had come to mean to me, and to thank her for giving Emma as a guide dog after puppy-walking her. That was the beginning of a correspondence by cassette, and of a friendship that continues to this day.

Through this correspondence I learned all sorts of little details about Emma. Paddy had her from the age of eight weeks, and she sent me a photograph taken at this time. Although I had to rely on other people's descriptions of the photograph it was splendid to have a picture of Emma as she was when she was first picked out of the litter to be a guide dog. She was already eighteen months old when I first met her, so of course I missed all her puppy ways, but to hear Paddy describe them on cassette was the best possible substitute. She said that Emma had always seemed a busy dog, was interested from the beginning in doing things constructively, and always gave the impression of having something on her mind. This confirmed what I knew of her.

On one cassette Paddy told me a story that I possibly found more amusing than she had at the time. One day Paddy planted some hundred and fifty bulbs in her garden. She had then gone indoors, leaving Emma still playing on the lawn. After about half an hour, Emma came in looking extremely pleased with herself. When Paddy happened to look out of the window a moment or so later, she was confronted with a huge pile of bulbs neatly stacked on the back doorstep. Emma had dug each one up with loving care and immense energy, and was thrilled to have been such a help in restoring them to their owner.

Before long, Paddy asked me to visit her in Yorkshire. They were having a small function to raise money for guide dogs at a local fete and she rightly thought I would like to go with Emma. Through our cassette correspondence, I felt I already knew Paddy, but I wondered if Emma would remember her. As we got off the coach I heard Paddy's voice greeting us, 'Hello, Sheila. How are you?' And it was the signal for Emma to go wild. She leaped all over Paddy, but although she was delighted to see her again, she kept coming back to me as if to say, 'Well, I'm pleased to be here, but I haven't forgotten that I'm your dog.'

Emma and I started to go to work together as soon as we were settled again. At that time I lived in Carlton, on one side of Nottingham, and I worked right over the other side, the Bulwell side of the city. I had to catch two buses, with a walk across the Market Square in the middle of Nottingham in between. The terminus for the first bus was at the bottom of our road, so that part was easy. Emma trotted down the road with her tail in the air – I could feel it brushing my hand as we went along – and, at the same time, I began to learn how sensitive it was possible to be, via the harness, to what she was doing. Through it I could tell whether her ears were up or down, whether she was turning her head left or right, and all sorts of little movements.

We found the stop, and from that moment Emma loved going on buses. It was not just the bus itself, however. One important factor was the admiration she received that morning, and every time we got on a bus henceforth: 'Oh, what a lovely dog. Oh, what a beautiful colour.' And so on. I could sense Emma basking in the glory. She had picked the second seat on the right for me. For some reason, this was the place she always chose on this particular bus. I sat down, and Emma went under the seat. Strangely, this was the only bus on which she had such a preference: it always had to be the same one. After we had been going to work together for about three weeks, we were nearing the bus one morning when I began to pick up the sound of a great commotion going on inside it. As we came alongside I could hear a woman's muffled shout: 'You'll have to get up you know. You can't sit there, I tell you it's Emma's seat. Come on – they'll be here in a minute.'

On other buses, Emma simply went for any empty seat, preferably – in the winter at least – one near the heaters. But since we normally travelled in the rush hour the buses, apart from our first one, were very often full, so she had to use a different technique. She would drag me along the aisle, nosing everyone else out of the way if there were standing passengers, decide on where she wanted us to sit, then stare at whoever was sitting there until they gave way. To be fair, they normally gave the seat up very quickly, and before the bus was in an uproar. This, of course, appealed to the exhibitionist in Emma. When she was sure she had got her audience, she would turn to me, lay her head across my knee, looking, I imagined, specially devoted and possibly a little pathetic. By this time the entire bus was hers.

But to get back to that first morning. When I walked into the office there was a reception committee waiting. While everyone said 'Hello' to me, they were clearly more interested in seeing what Emma was like. Emma once again responded with great delight, and when I had taken her harness off, took it round, her tail wagging, to show everyone in turn.

So she was a hit straight away, and when the others had gone she inspected her basket, played for a while with a rubber toy I had brought with me to occupy her, then settled down. The telephone had already started going, and soon it was like old times – with the tremendous difference of that reassuring sleeping form under my desk. The morning went on, and in a lull, thinking what a good quiet dog Emma was being, I put my hand down to pat her head. But, where her head should have been, there was nothing. I felt round in a wider circle. Emma had disappeared! I immediately got up and went to feel if my office door was open; sure enough, it was. I called her. No response. All sorts of anxieties began to crowd in on me. Had she got out? What if she had gone into the street? What if she were lost … what … then I heard the sound of paws coming down the corridor. Thank goodness. In came Emma. 'Emma,' I said, 'where *have you* been?' Her reply was to push something into my lap. I did not want to believe my fingers. It was a purse. I was horrified. 'Emma! Where did you get that from?' Her reply this time was to do her tattoo bit, bouncing up and down on her forelegs, and swishing me furiously with her tail. The message was clear: 'How about that for brilliance! I've brought you somebody's purse.' Fleetingly, the thought of a four-legged Artful Dodger came to mind. I took the purse from her, and hoped that someone would come and claim it, and accept my excuses.

The owner concerned eventually found out what had happened, and came to claim the purse. But no one would believe that I had not taught Emma to perform the trick, which did nothing to ease my mind about the prospect of the afternoon, or indeed of continuing to work for Industrial Pumps. It was a relief to take Emma out of the office for a run in the local park. This was something I had decided I must do every day. Since she worked hard it was only fair that she should have a free run whenever possible.

I sat myself on a bench with my sandwiches, let her off the lead, and she went charging across the grass. I soon heard barking in the distance, and recognised Emma. But every so often she would come back to me, touch my hands with her nose, and then scamper off again. It was something that she never failed to do whenever we went to the park from then on. She was reassuring me: 'I'm here, and I haven't forgotten you.'

That afternoon I sat down at the switchboard, and, in between calls, waited uneasily for the sound of Emma bringing me another gift. But she settled down and slept, and after that did not bring any more presents – at least, not in the office. Perhaps it was her way of making her mark, and returning her welcome. Whatever it was, I was pleased it was over.

The first week went by very happily. Travelling to and from work, in fact, became easier every day. I did not have to give Emma all the lefts and rights in the Square because she soon began to take me straight to the right road and across to the forty-three bus stop. I started to appreciate, and this was something that established itself firmly as time went on, that Emma had only to take any route once and she knew it. I had no sooner discovered this than I found there was a drawback in having such an intelligent dog.

About the middle of the second week we set off for work as usual. I merely said to Emma that we were going to work, and, by now, knew she could do this without any corrections or promptings. We got our first bus, and reached the Market Square. Everything was fine. But when we got to the first road to cross in the Square, Emma sat down instead of going forward. I listened for traffic, and when I thought it was clear, told her to go forward. But she would not move. She simply continued to sit. I could not understand what was going on. I thought that perhaps I had misjudged the traffic, so when it was quiet I told her again. Still she would not go forward. Instead, she got up and turned right, and started taking me along the pavement. 'Emma,' I said, rather desperately, as I was being dragged along, 'where are you taking me? Where's the bus stop? Come on. Bus stop …' But no, she would not listen, or if she did listen she certainly did not take any notice. We went on, across a road, made a sharp left turn, and crossed another road. Then she sat down again. I had no idea where we were. I had completely lost my sense of direction, and was utterly confused about the pattern I had to keep in my mind in order to reach the bus stop; this was the equivalent of the checks that sighted people, probably unconsciously, make when they are getting from A to B: right at St Mary's Church, past WH Smith, left at the Royal Oak, and so on.

I was not only disappointed in Emma, but slightly upset and annoyed with her as well. 'Emma,' I said crossly, 'we shall be late for work.' How do you tell the boss that it was the dog who made you late? Thinking back, it must have looked a rather comic scene to anyone passing by. 'Excuse me,' I said as the next foot-steps approached, 'can you tell me how to get to the forty-three bus stop, please?' There was a silence for a second or two, during which time I thought: 'They don't know, we really are lost.' Then a man's voice, obviously puzzled, said, 'Forty-three bus stop? You're *at* the forty-three bus stop. Your dog's at the foot of the post.' I was relieved, astonished and utterly baffled. We got on the bus when it came along, and I put the incident out of my mind. Until the following morning.

This time Emma went left instead of right, crossed another road, turned right; crossed a further road, walked along and sat down. We were at the forty-three bus stop again. I was unnerved, but by now getting used to the feeling. At work, I asked Carol, a friend who I knew came to the office via the Market Square, if there were any roadworks on the route I had originally mapped out. She said no, and no new building either, or any kind of obstruction.

I was totally at a loss. I thought and thought, and then the only possible explanation came to me: Emma, having learned a route, became bored with having to follow it every day. So she invented variations. From then on she found a series of routes round the Market

Square quite independently of any guidance from me, and chose one of them every day. I soon became resigned to this and got up ten minutes earlier just to allow for Emma possibly making a mistake. But, of course, she never did.

5

Anita

B<small>Y NOW</small> I was learning that Emma gave me a certain freedom not only to go where I liked but also to do what I liked. The limits were not as narrow as might be imagined. All sorts of subjects fascinated me and I decided to enrol in an evening class called Writer's Craft. It was through this that I met Anita.

During one of the tea breaks at the class I heard a warm, friendly voice saying, 'Hello, and aren't you a beautiful dog?' And then to me, 'Do you mind if I talk to your dog? I've never met a guide dog before. She really is a beautiful colour.' The owner of the voice, which had a strong Yorkshire accent, eventually introduced herself as Anita. And this was the start of a very true friendship – all because of Emma. Anita was nineteen, the same age as I was, and she had come to take a job in Nottingham. I gathered later that she was attractive and had a good figure and short, dark hair. As the weeks went by I came to look forward to meeting her at the classes. She was interested in writing short stories, and I was trying to write poetry. We always chatted at the break, and one night I asked her what she did at the weekends.

'I go back to Hull quite a bit,' she said, 'but this coming weekend I'm going riding.'

Riding! My heart skipped a beat. It was something I had always yearned to try, something I had heard so much about from girlfriends. But my mother had always resolutely forbidden it. In my mind I could hear her words, 'Certainly not, Sheila. No, I won't entertain the idea for a minute.'

But now Anita's mention of this forbidden activity gave me a thought – and my mother need never know. 'How marvellous,' I said, 'Would you take me?'

From the tone of her voice Anita was obviously very surprised. 'Take you? Would you really want to, Sheila? I mean, wouldn't you be scared? I mean … because you can't see properly?' This was a reaction I was not prepared for, strange as it may seem. I had never thought of my blindness as an obstacle. 'Never even thought about it,' I said.

'Well,' said Anita, 'I'll book a ride for you too. I'll phone you at work tomorrow.'

I waited for her call with some excitement. But it was not until the afternoon that the phone rang, and Anita's voice betrayed that something had gone wrong. 'Sheila, I don't know how to say this. I've been in touch with the stable, and half a dozen others as well. They won't take you. They all refused point-blank ... I'm afraid it's because you can't see.'

There was a pause while I let this sink in. Then she added, 'And I've cancelled my ride as well.'

'Oh, Anita,' I said, 'why did you do that?'

'Because if they won't have you, I don't want to go either. Why should they discriminate just because you can't see?'

Her kindness lightened my gloom at the thought of no one accepting me. The gesture was typical of her – warm-hearted and unselfish. Even so, I felt guilty about spoiling her weekend and said so.

'No, Sheila,' she said. 'It doesn't matter a bit. Anyway, we'll get you on a horse somehow, even if it means trying to pretend that you can see.'

The switchboard buzzed again within minutes. It was Anita, with a triumphant note this time in her no-nonsense voice. 'I've booked rides for both of us.'

I was thrilled. And apprehensive. 'How are we going to do it? How can we hide the fact that I can't see? They're bound to notice, and then you'll get into hot water. And something else: what about Emma? They'll know she's a guide dog because of her harness.'

'Leave it all to me,' said Anita. 'We'll think of something. And I'm sure we can get someone to look after Emma and hide her harness.'

I could not get over her persistence. She was doing all this just for me. When the weekend came I put on a sweater, and, because I had no proper riding gear, my oldest slacks. They were the subject of critical comment from my mother, but I prudently let the subject rest. Emma and I met Anita as arranged, and as we took a bus to the stable, she told me what she had planned.

'I've got it all worked out. We're going to meet a friend of mine who will take charge of Emma's harness just outside the stable. Then we'll link arms and get you to your horse, and I'll make it clear that I'm helping you up because you've never ridden before. When you get up on your horse, I'll tell you what to do, and we'll keep talking to one another all the time after we set off, so you'll know exactly where I am.'

It sounded fine. But I could not help feeling a slight panic already stirring in me. At the same time I knew I could not back out. I thought, 'I must bluff for Anita's sake.'

We met Anita's friend and gave her Emma's harness, while Emma herself accompanied the three of us on a lead. Then, in the stable yard, the tight feeling inside gripped me. I could hear all sorts of voices. I felt sure someone was going to come up and say, 'You can't see! What are you doing trying to ride one of our horses?'

But everyone was too busy with his own mount to bother with me, and I was heaved up on to the back of my horse, after some fumbling for the stirrup. Anita had brought him to me, and said he was called Rocky. I sat up on his back, feeling very strange and hissed, 'Now what, what do I do?'

'Don't worry,' came the reply as I heard her alongside me. 'Give me your hands. This is how you put your fingers and thumbs round the reins. Like that. That's it. No, thumbs outwards. That's it. Now hold on, and when we're ready to go, just gently dig your heels in his flanks ... not too hard ...'

So we moved along, and I heard Anita just behind me, keeping up a running commentary: 'Isn't that a fantastic old oak tree... What's Rocky like, Sheila? ... He's very Roman-nosed isn't he? ... Isn't that lovely down there?' and so on, in order to reassure me of her presence.

All went well, and I was feeling quite relaxed as we trotted gently along. I was imagining that I was Maid Marian in Sherwood Forest sedately riding to meet Robin Hood, when suddenly something must have frightened Rocky. He half-reared, then took off with me at a brisk canter. I was petrified. I dropped the reins and grabbed the saddle and hung on.

The wind rushed by my face. I heard Anita shouting, 'Pull your reins back. Sit back in the saddle.' All her instructions were to no avail. I was carried on helplessly, as never before through my daylight world of darkness, bumping up and down, just hanging on, powerless.

Then, as capriciously as he'd started, Rocky slackened his pace. He came to a halt and put his head down, and I heard him tearing up grass, chomping it in his teeth. But that was the only sound there was. A new fear set in. I had completely lost my sense of direction. I should never have done it. I thought, 'Now they're bound to find out I'm blind. And they'll blame Anita.'

At that moment I heard hooves again, and Anita's voice: 'Go on, Sheila, make him move. Dig your heels in, don't just sit there.' At last, after some prodding and persuasion and more advice from Anita, we got Rocky to move. When we returned to the stable, no one even suspected that I was blind. All I overheard was: 'Trust Rocky to take off like that. Rather her than me. I reckon she did well to stay on.'

We had got away with it! And, despite the sensational behaviour of Rocky, I had to admit that I had enjoyed it, and from then on, when we could, Anita and I used to go riding together.

One day Anita invited me back to her flat. While we were drinking tea, she said suddenly, 'You know, I don't very much like this flat, Sheila. It's terribly small and cramped. I'd love something bigger, but everything's so expensive. I went to a lovely one the other day. It was fabulous – big sitting room and separate bedroom. Not like here, where you have to make the bed do for a sofa during the day, and where the kitchen's no bigger than a cupboard. If I could get someone to share with me, then I might be able to afford it. But I suppose it's all a dream – like getting my short stories published!'

We both laughed. But her remarks had planted a seed in my mind. I had already decided that I would like to go out into the world and be independent, now that I had Emma to guide me. At home I did my share of the household tasks, and I knew I was capable of doing the same elsewhere. Yet, independence had never been more than a dream.

What would Anita say if I suggested that I might be the one to share with her and solve her problem? I deliberated for a moment and said, 'How about sharing with me?'

Her reaction was more than I had dared hope for. 'Oh, Sheila, what a terrific idea!'

But I thought I had better find out if she realised all the implications. 'Do you *really* think it would be a good idea? What about Emma, for instance?'

'Well, you couldn't come without Emma. I just took that for granted.'

'Ah. What I really mean is … Doesn't the fact that I can't see put you off a bit?'

'Put me off? No, of course not. You get along at home quite well. Why shouldn't you do the same sharing with me?'

It was a tantalising, enormous idea. Yet I did not

want her to rush into something she might regret and, to be honest, it would mean so many changes in my life that I thought we should not decide there and then. I suggested we consider the whole business overnight. Anita agreed, but as she saw Emma and me to the door she said, 'I'm certain I know what the answer's going to be.'

There was, however, a possible complication that I had forgotten to mention during our exciting discussion: Tiss. Tiss was my ginger cat.

One of the first things I had wanted to do after I got Emma home from Leamington was to buy a kitten, in the hope that Emma would gradually overcome her dislike of cats. We went along to the local pet shop and after the man had described all the kittens he had, I thought a ginger tom sounded the nicest. So this small bundle of fur was removed from the cage and placed in my hands: warm and tiny, its heart pounding. Emma apparently looked at him quite thoughtfully, and I felt her put her nose up to him in my hands. She did not run a mile, and he did not spit at her. So he was the one. He was lovely, but grew into a strange cat, slightly schizophrenic.

Tiss (just a nickname that stuck) came into our home a small fluffy ball of good nature and friendliness. He took to Emma, and she to him, although for the first few days she used to mistake him for a furry, animated toy, and would pick him up, so I was told, and throw him about. But he would wash Emma's ears, lick her nose with his rough little tongue and purr, and they would sit at the fireside together. I imagined them as a picture of bliss.

Then Tiss began to show the other side of his nature: he would wait on the arm of a chair and when Emma passed would leap off and swing on her ear. Emma never protested, or seemed to mind other teasings that Tiss got up to.

He was so silent about the place that I could never hear where he was and was afraid of treading on him until I bought him a collar and little bell. But he soon learned how to move without tinkling the bell. Tricks apart, he seemed to worship Emma, and despite the dislike she had always shown for cats, she made an exception for Tiss. He in turn would never go to sleep without Emma, and this he did by curling up on top of her in the dog bed.

Tiss, therefore, was a consideration when it came to deciding about moving into a flat with Anita. But I finally thought, 'Why not?' Anita said she did not mind sharing with a Labrador and a ginger tom, so we started hunting round the house agents and the streets of Nottingham for a flat.

First, however, I had to break the idea to my mother. She worried about me anyway, so I did not anticipate an over-enthusiastic reaction. Yet I hoped she would approve because one of her great principles was that blind people should be part of the sighted world as far as they could. She was washing up when I explained the plan to her, and, partly because she was hard of hearing, and partly because of the noise of suds and crockery, I thought at first she hadn't heard me. Then she said, 'Are you sure you want to do this?'

'Yes mum, quite sure.'

'Well, I mean, are you certain you'll be able to manage? It's a big break.'

'Yes, I'm certain I can do it. And it really is a chance to be independent.'

At that moment, Graham came in from work. He had a job as a piano-tuner, although his great passion was playing the guitar. When he heard what I was proposing, he said, 'I think it's great. You'll cope, won't you, Sheila?'

My mother was silent, and I sensed that she was torn between natural maternal anxiety, and wanting me to put into practice what she had always taught me. Finally she said, 'Well, you know best what you can do, Sheila, and if you want any help or things don't work out, then you can always have a bed here in the back room.'

Actually finding a flat wasn't so easy. The difficulties mainly arose not because of a shortage of accommodation, but because I was blind. So many times we turned up for an appointment, and, as Anita told me after-wards, the face of the prospective landlord or landlady dropped when they realised I could not see. What kind of liability, I wonder, did they expect me to be? Would I blunder round and smash the furniture, overflow the bath and bring the plaster down, or simply cause the entire house to go up in flames? Those that did not mind me took exception to Emma or Tiss, or both. It seemed hopeless. Then, after nearly three months, and countless disappointments, we finally found a small self-contained flat. It was in Peel Street, a row of large nineteenth-century country houses, rather decayed, near the old Nottingham Victoria station which has now been pulled down to make way for a shopping precinct. It was a three-roomed flat which smelled rather musty, and was furnished with a minimum of creaky chairs and rickety tables. There was a kitchen converted from what may well have been a boot cupboard in better days, and we were grateful for the handbasin and a cooker which Anita described to me as a genuine relic from the galley of the ark.

Anita was the practical one of the household. As soon as we moved into the flat she said, 'We've got to be absolutely fair and straight down the line with expenses. I think we ought to have a kitty, particularly for the food. I'll get a tin and you put three pounds in, and I'll do the same.'

We were just deciding this important point when we had our first visitor. It was Graham, who had brought some cases of clothes for me. He did a tour of inspection and gave his verdict. 'Not bad,' he said, 'not bad at all. But it needs a bit of brightening up. And you haven't got a clock.'

'Yes, I have,' I said. 'It's in the bedroom.'

'Oh, that. That's your braille alarm clock. I mean a clock that other people can see. Anita will want to tell the time too.'

The following day Graham was back with a kitchen clock which he screwed into the wall for us, as a house-warming present. It was so characteristic of him to choose something that would link me with the sighted world.

There were other flats in the house, and we were soon on speaking terms with our neighbours, but for a variety of reasons never managed to hit it off with the member of the Fire Brigade who lived immediately below us in the basement flat. It was partly my fault. Anita used to go away a lot at weekends to stay with her parents and see her boyfriend in Hull, and she left me in charge. This made me nervous at first, but I soon got used to running the place on my own, with some help from Emma. It seemed an enormous step towards becoming more independent. One of the first weekends that Anita went away, before I had become absolutely used to the place, I decided to take the small kitchen waste bin down to the dustbins outside. These were reached through the front garden, down a little passageway, through a gate, and were ranged in a row next to the rockery kept by the fireman. Emma came with me, although she was not on her harness. She might have saved me if she had been; but there seemed no point, since we were not going for a proper outing. Somehow, a brick had been left in the middle of the passageway. On harness, Emma would immediately have taken me round it. As it was, she merely stood by and watched. I tripped over the brick and let go of the rubbish all over the fireman, who had just emerged from his flat, covering him with cigarette ends, banana skins and other assorted oddments.

Our relationship did not improve the following Saturday. Anita was once again away. I had decided that the kitchen needed a good clean, particularly the waste bin that had figured so prominently in the previous week's episode. I boiled two kettles, filled the bin with water and disinfectant, and left it for an hour below the washbasin. When I went to empty it, it felt ominously light. I put my hand in it. No water. How was I to know that there had been a hole in the plastic? Or that the water would seep through the floor and into the fireman's kitchen? Things were never the same again.

The most bizarre mistake I made occurred one weekend after we had been at the flat for a few months, and I had become quite used to running it. In addition to Emma and Tiss, the animal population of the household had recently been increased by Anita's purchase of a pair of pet mice, called Ilk and Moke. I suppose they were sold as tame mice, although I would have sued the pet shop under the Trade Descriptions Act. It was impossible to put a hand in their cage and bring it out unscratched. Tiss loathed them. When Anita went away I used to have to feed these small sharp-clawed monsters.

One weekend I had them in their cage on the kitchen table, and had piled books on top so that Tiss could not leap on to their roof and stare and hiss down at them. On the Sunday morning I got up and went with Emma into the kitchen to make a cup of tea. I knew I had left the matches on the table, and felt round for them. But then I heard something move near my hand. I almost had heart failure. I put out my hand for the matchbox, and there was the sound again: small claws. I was petrified. It had to be a mouse.

I went hot and cold. I thought I must have let one of them out when I was feeding them the previous day. What would Anita think? What if it escaped? Anita would be bound to think Tiss had caught it. How could I get it back? I stood there in my dressing gown dithering, and then had a brainwave. Much as I loathed the idea, I had to catch it, and I knew there was a tin handy. I felt for this empty tin, and brought it up to the edge of the table. There I waited, quite still, for minutes on end: it must have been a weird sight. Suddenly I heard a movement. Then, sure enough, I felt the mouse – was it Ilk? Or was it Moke? I didn't care. Anyway, I felt him on the tin, and quickly got him in and clapped my hand over the top, at the same time opening the cage. Before he could scratch or bite I had him back inside and crashed the cage door to.

It took me several cups of tea to recover. But at least I could face Anita on her return. When she did come back, late that evening, one of the first things she did was to go and inspect her mice.

'Sheila,' she said, 'my mice.'

'Yes,' I said haplessly, my heart turning over (had I let them *both* out when I opened the cage?)

'Sheila, what happened? There are three!'

'Three?'

'Yes, *three*, my white ones and a grey one.'

Grey one! I immediately knew what had happened. Covered in confusion I explained. We collapsed with laughter. It occurred to me that it was quite the reverse of Three Blind Mice!

Normally, however, things went reasonably smoothly, particularly when Anita was there. She was great fun to live with, and I was well aware how lucky I was to have my own flat, which is more than many sighted people have. We used to laugh a lot, and I was often amused by some of the Yorkshire expressions she came out with. One cold November day I had chosen a rather flimsy dress to wear.

'You can't wear that,' Anita said.

'Why not?'

'You'll catch King Cough if you go out in that.'

'King Cough? What's that?'

'Didn't your mother ever tell you? I don't know! King Cough's three times worse than any other cough, and you catch your death of it.'

Impressed by the idea and possible power of King Cough, I changed into something warmer.

I imagine that when Anita first asked me if I would share with her, it must have occurred to her that there would be disadvantages in living with me. For my part it was difficult to admit that I could not do everything a sighted person could, yet I was determined to show that the handicap was not as bad as might have been imagined. In fact, I think I may possibly have surprised Anita by how much I could do, even though I was blind. It meant a great deal of hard work and concentration. Still, we persevered. I would do the hoovering, while Anita dusted. Sometimes, above the noise of the vacuum cleaner, I would hear her laughing. I'd switch off and say, 'Now what are you laughing at?' And she would giggle. 'Well, you've been over that bit of carpet about six times – and there's a huge bit that still needs doing only two inches away.' So off I would go again, and wait for the next correction, until finally I would have the entire carpet clean.

The food cupboard in the flat was a source of amusement after shopping expeditions. If I was in charge I would buy only the food I wanted for the next twenty-four hours, because too many tins and packets would be confusing. Each evening I would buy the supplies we wanted for supper, breakfast and tea, and I would try to keep various foodstuffs separate in the cupboard: a shelf for vegetables, part of another one for tins of fruit, another part for tins of dog meat, and so on. Sometimes my planning did not work out. Emma, I think, very much enjoyed best tinned casserole steak one night, and I did not pursue what happened to the tin of pet food she should have had. With packets and jars, one way of identifying the contents was of course by smell. So if I wanted marmalade, I had to take each jar out of the cupboard, unscrew the top, and sniff what was inside. With jam, pickles, and so on this was fairly easy, if laborious; it also developed my sense of smell. But with things such as salt or sugar, I just had to wet my finger and taste – and sometimes got quite a surprise.

One of the activities that really fascinated Anita was my cooking. 'I just don't understand,' she would say, 'how you can cook.' In fact, it is not as difficult as it may sound. I tried to explain to her that whether you have sight or not, a great deal of cooking is actually done by touch. If you are boiling potatoes, you put a fork in them to test if they are done. If you are roasting a joint of meat, you put a skewer in it from time to time. Admittedly, people with sight do not rely on this entirely, but it may explain why cooking was not impossible for me. I could use the cooker itself by feel, and in addition I had a braille temperature gauge fitted to the oven. The only thing I really disliked was frying, because the fat tended to spit, and, obviously, I could not use a skewer to test whether a fried egg was done or not. The other sense I used was smell, which was possibly of more value in preventing over-cooking than in cooking itself. After we had been at the flat a little time I think I convinced Anita that I was capable of pulling my weight.

I had to rely on Anita a great deal for dress sense. We were a similar shape and size and I sometimes borrowed her clothes. She helped me a lot. It is very difficult to pick the right clothes if you can't see the colours, and can only touch the garments to get an idea of the material and style. When I went into a shop in the days before I shared with Anita it was very often a case of 'Never mind the quality, feel the width.' But with her advice it was marvellous to be able to wear clothes that I knew were fashionable. She would come along with me to the shops, or, if I went with Emma, I would take the outfit on approval, try it on back at the flat and ask Anita's honest opinion. 'No, it's just not you,' she might say, or, 'No, I don't think so. It makes you look about ninety.' So back to the shop the clothes would go. I suppose I was really wearing clothes that Anita herself liked, rather than those that I might like if I could have seen, but I still found it all very liberating. Anita, after all, was my age and kept up with the fashion magazines, and for the first time in my life, I felt I too was a reasonably decorative part of the fashion scene.

As well as helping with my clothes, Anita was also able to tell me if my hair looked right. She was my looking glass. But, over and above that, the best thing about her was the feeling that she was treating me as a paid-up member of the human race. She had a great sense of honesty, and there was never any suggestion of making embarrassing allowances for the fact that I could not see.

That said, there was one thing I had to be wary of with her, and that was when we used to do our shopping together. It was pleasant for Emma to have Anita take over guiding me when we went into town. It meant Emma did not have her harness on, and off-duty could go on a lead like any other dog going for a walk. But it was not always so good for me, because I would occasionally trip or collide painfully with a lamp post, and Anita would say, 'Oh, Sheila, I'm so sorry, I was looking in a shop window, I didn't see that.' In the end, I am afraid, I went back to relying entirely on Emma, even when we all went out together.

It was while I was at the flat I came to realise how close a bond had grown up between Emma and me, and not only on my side. When I first had Emma, she was never less than splendid in her work, despite her independence in choosing her own routes, and so on. But I got the impression that, although I needed her, she did not really need me. She would look after me when we were going along the street, but indoors at the house where we first lived she would never bark when there was a knock on the door. She had no protective instinct towards me. Once we had settled in at the flat, when, after the upheaval of moving and despite the change of surroundings, she knew we were still together, her attitude gradually changed. We began to spend a great deal of time on our own, and of course Emma was with me twenty-four hours a day. She would follow me about, which she had not done before, and never let me out of her sight – even in the bathroom. Moreover, not only did we begin to walk with the same pace and kind of step, but we seemed to develop an instinct for knowing one another's thoughts – a sort of telepathy. It may sound incredible, but it was perfectly true.

Industrial Pumps had moved their premises to Colwick and I used to do the shopping for the weekend at lunchtime on Fridays in a little area called Netherfield. Emma always knew it was Friday, and I never had to say anything; she would simply take me to Netherfield, whereas on every other day we went for our usual walk. One Monday, however, I wanted to take my watch to be repaired, and the nearest jeweller was in Netherfield. I had never been to the jeweller's before, and as I did not know where it was exactly, I got full directions from Carol. Since it was a Monday, I assumed Emma would think we were going for our usual outing, and for some reason I did not tell her that the plan had changed. We went out of the office as usual and to the main road. But instead of our customary Monday route, she unhesitatingly carried on over the bridge, turned right into the shopping centre at Netherfield, took me on for two blocks, entered a shop and sat down. I was astounded. We were in the jeweller's. How could she possibly have known we were going to our usual Friday area on a Monday? Even more astonishing, how could she possibly have known we were going to that shop? I certainly hadn't said a word to her about it.

'How did you *know*, Emma?' I said. And I could hear her tail beating on the floor. 'Oh, all right,' I said, 'I give in. I'll never try to keep you in the dark again.' And I never did.

6

Don

WHILE WE WERE at the flat, our local radio station, Radio Nottingham, came on the air for the first time. One of the programmes introduced, *Wednesday Club*, was specially for blind people. It was run by George Miller, who was a newspaper reporter and blind himself. It always astonished me that someone who could not see was able to do this kind of work. Yet George not only made his living from journalism; he did the job magnificently. One day, he got in touch with me to ask if I would go on the *Wednesday Club* programme and talk about guide dogs. I said I would, but I did not very much like the idea of sitting in front of a microphone and giving a lot of facts and figures about guide dogs: I didn't think the audience could be held like that. A better way of putting over just what guide dogs can do would be to have some sort of practical demonstration involving Emma and me. So I suggested having a bet that we could get from any one part of Nottingham to another faster than a sighted person.

George laughed and said they would think about it. A day or so later he rang back and said OK to the idea, and told me that Tony Church, the producer, would be the one with whom I would have the bet. He made it quite clear, however, that everyone at Radio Nottingham thought I was out of my mind, and that Emma and I had as much chance of winning as a three-legged horse in the Derby.

Tony Church mapped out a route that he told me he would disclose on the day of the recording. Emma and I accordingly turned up outside the Radio Nottingham studios. Tony was there to meet us, with his tape recorder and microphone.

'Well, this is the famous Emma, this is the dog that's going to beat me, is it?'

'Yes, it is,' I said, while I imagined Emma giving him a piercing look of confirmation that this was indeed what was going to happen.

'All right,' said Tony, 'do you know Trinity Square?' Trinity Square? This was great.

'Yes,' I said. 'Very well.'

'Well, now, whereabouts in Trinity Square would you like to head for?'

I thought for a moment, and then decided. 'The forty-nine bus stop,' I said.

'Right,' said Tony, and off we went. We had to cross quite a few busy main roads in order to reach this particular square, and to begin with I could hear Tony behind me, using his tape recorder to give a commentary on what was going on, though before long his voice was drowned by the traffic sounds.

Emma and I pounded on, Emma seeming more agile and nimble than ever, and at last we reached Trinity Square, and the bus station winning post. Tony did not arrive until a few minutes later. Rather out of breath and somewhat stunned, he said, 'Congratulations, and apologies. You were right, and we were wrong.'

It was not until I heard the tape played back in the studio that I learned what had happened: it was no doubt entertaining for the listeners, but it also enlightened me about the way Emma worked. In the first place, I was surprised at the number of obstacles that she had taken me round about which I had known nothing. She had also taken me across a zebra crossing. I had stopped while Emma had sat down, and we waited until I could hear the traffic draw up. I remember at this point that Emma had got up first and crossed the road. What I did not know was that a bus had pulled up at the crossing, and the driver had leaned out of his cab and waved Emma over. As we reached the other side, Tony had come panting up. But the bus moved on at that moment and left him stranded on the opposite end of the crossing. He then ran along that side of the road, trying to keep up with us. When he did finally cross and catch us up, he trod on Emma's tail, which did not go down at all well. Then, trying to get across the next road, the same sort of thing happened again. The traffic waited for us, but not for Tony. As we reached Trinity Square, we were well in front, and Emma, according to the tape, had time to stop and look in a shop window that seemed to interest her. It had a huge notice: 'Sale On'.

That programme for Radio Nottingham was the beginning of my friendship with George Miller. He was an extremely likeable man, full of vivacity and zest for life. From then on he often used to ring me up and discuss the *Wednesday Club* programmes. He was very keen on helping other blind people, and rightly considered the whole venture a worthwhile contribution in this direction. Sometimes he rang up and chatted about a piece of news concerning the blind; or he consulted me about guide dog work.

One evening, George telephoned and said he had a friend with him, someone called Don Hocken. Would I like a word with him? Don was in the same room and could hear the conversation through the speaker that had been fitted on to George's telephone to leave his hands free for his braille machine. Don came on the line and passed the time of day, and if it is possible to fall in love immediately over the telephone, I certainly did.

When Don told me what his work was (he was a chiropodist) I'm afraid I laughed: I thought of someone condemned to a fate of endlessly cutting other people's toenails. He put me right, however. It was, he said, rather more complicated than that. But, more important, he did not seem to mind my laughter one bit, although I later learned how much his work meant to him, and what a close interest he took in his patients.

Don was fond of dogs and had heard from George about Emma, so we chatted away for some time about her, and poor George hardly got a word in at all. When we had rung off I could not get over the sound of Don's soft, deep voice and the conversation kept replaying itself in my mind. I discovered afterwards that Don had first met George as a patient and on the day of the first consultation, not realising George was blind, Don had put his groping approach to the surgery door down to excess alcohol! They struck up a friendship and George had been helping Don with some of his own writing efforts.

A few evenings later George rang again, and Don was there too. I was thrilled. When he came on the line I wondered what he looked like, but, strangely, I felt on a par with him in a way that would have been impossible if we had been introduced face to face. Because we had 'met' on the telephone he was equally unaware of my appearance. Then he told me that he had been invited to the Open Day the following Saturday at Radio Nottingham, and suddenly I felt nervous. I had also been invited, and, after he had rung off, I wondered whether I dared go. I simply did not want to face the fact that if he had illusions they might dissolve when he saw me. Moreover, I never believed that a sighted man could really be attracted to a woman who was blind. But I thought it over, and in the end my curiosity won. I decided I would go.

I remember that day in August 1968 so well. I went right through my wardrobe wondering what to wear. I finally chose my best green dress, and newest shoes: I could never wear high heels because they led to too many difficulties on kerbs and gratings; but fashion by then was getting round to the flatter heels I had to wear, and as it happened, I had just bought a pair of shoes that were considered very smart. I had been to the hairdresser, and I kept asking Anita: 'Do I look all right? Is my hair OK? Do I really look presentable? What do you honestly think?' Anita kept reassuring me: 'Oh, Sheila, you look fine, you really do, don't be silly.'

But it was impossible for me to compare myself accurately with other people and therefore judge for myself what I looked like. As a result, I always felt that I could not be as well dressed as any one else, or that my hair could never look as good as theirs. When people said, as they often did, 'You look nice', I could never be sure that they were not making allowances somehow for the fact that I was blind.

At last, after these great preparations, Emma and I set off. Emma knew I was excited, because she pushed herself forward in her harness and wagged her tail as we went along. I told her all about Don. 'He sounds very nice, Emma,' I said, 'but I don't know what he'll make of us, I really don't.' Emma went on wagging her tail, but the further we went, the more nervous I became. Silly, but there it was. I could not analyse it to myself at the time, but this meeting seemed so very, very important and special.

We arrived at Radio Nottingham, and, once inside, I could hear a big crowd. Eventually I managed to get someone to find George for me. They were away for a bit, then I heard George's voice. We went to sit in a corner and chat, while all sorts of people came up to talk to him, and finished up having a conversation with Emma. In the middle of it all, I heard this unmistakable voice, talking some distance away. I thought, 'I wonder if he's seen me? I wonder what he thinks? Perhaps he's seen me and doesn't want to come over and meet us after all.' Then I could pick out what he was saying. He was talking to a girl with a young, attractive voice, and he said, 'The last time I saw you, you were in bed.' I was astonished, and thought: 'Well, would you believe it? He's just one of these characters who sweep girls off their feet, and straight into bed.' I felt terribly let down. Then I heard more of the conversation. It transpired that while he had been visiting his mother in hospital, this girl had been in the next bed!

At last, I heard him say goodbye to her, then there was the approach of footsteps, and the same voice, much nearer, said, 'Hello, Sheila.' In the same instant I knew he was smiling. Emma got up and gave him a huge welcome. He patted her and made a great fuss of her, but it was to me he quickly turned his attention. We sat down and began talking, and it was as if we had known each other for years. He described the studio in detail to me, the control panels, the double glazing, and everything about the surroundings and the people who were there. But it was not the description in itself that was marvellous – which it was – but the fact that Don knew I was cut off, and had immediately set about doing what he could to put this right by telling me all about what was going on.

'Would you like to come round the studio with me?' he asked eventually. I said I would, and was then surprised and delighted when he didn't immediately clutch at my arm and try to drag me round. Instead, he offered his arm for me to put my hand round, which is the best and easiest way to guide a blind person. He was not a bit embarrassed, and when we got to the control panel he insisted on my feeling all the dials and buttons.

'This is the control panel, Sheila: feel the control here; this is the window that looks out over the studio ...' Don seemed to have an instinctive grasp of how to make things come alive to someone who was blind. I felt completely relaxed and happy with him.

Later on in the afternoon he suggested to George that we all went to have some tea together (and by tea, I mean the kind of high tea we have in Nottingham, something more substantial than thin cucumber sandwiches). At first I did not much like the idea as I did not want to let myself down in front of Don when everything was so marvellous. I tried to make excuses that we really had to be getting back home. But he would not listen. 'Come on,' he said, 'I know a really nice place just up the road.' Finally he persuaded me, and Emma and I set off in front of George, who was being guided by Don. He had told me exactly where the restaurant was, and we arrived a little in front of them, which was pleasing, because I wanted to show that with Emma's guidance I was well able to cope.

Once inside, and having got permission for Emma to come in (always a problem in restaurants, and not one that the magic words 'guide dog' would necessarily solve), she curled up under the table and Don thoughtfully described the surroundings, including the decorations, carpets and curtains, and made the place vivid for me. We ordered steak. Don offered to cut it up for me. As always I refused, and later paid for this small show of independence. On the second occasion I got my fork to my mouth with nothing on it, I heard Don laugh, and say: 'You've missed again.' I was so embarrassed, I blushed from my toes to the roots of my hair. I wanted him to accept me as a normal person. Yet his laughter had no unkindness in it, and somehow his laughing it off in this way did make things easier in the end.

After the meal, Don drove Emma and me back to Peel Street. As we said goodbye outside the flat, just before he got back into the car, he handed me something. I felt it. It was a rose, and I suppose he had taken it out of his buttonhole. When I got in I put the rose in a vase, and cherished it. I kept it long after the bloom had gone; I never wanted to throw it away.

In the days that followed I would sometimes touch the rose in its vase which I had in my bedroom, and I kept going over the details of that Saturday in my mind. At the same time I had an uneasy feeling that I would never hear from Don again, that it had been a lovely day, and that was it. In my imagination he was tall and fair with a moustache. I knew he was tall because his voice came from above me, and I knew he was quite broad-shouldered from taking his arm on the tour of the studio. I was quite glad that Anita had not been there, and there was no one to give me his or her description of Don, because I always preferred the people of my imagination to the way they were described by others.

A few days went by, and I was beginning to think my fears about his not getting in touch again were right, when a voice that I instantly recognised came over the switchboard. I knew Don would not be ringing to order our latest model sewage pump. He wanted to take me out that evening. That evening! I was so excited that for the rest of the afternoon there was a high percentage of wrong calls to the wrong extensions all over the office.

On the way home I told Emma all about it. By that time, I had mentioned Don's name to her so often that she was quite familiar with it, and wagged her tail in reply. I think she was looking forward to the outing. Anita was still at work when we got back to the flat, so there was only Emma to share my excitement. I remember feeling the warmth of the sun in my bedroom as I started to change, and thinking how the world suddenly seemed to have become a warm and marvellous place.

As we went out that summer evening, which seemed more scented than any other evening I could remember, I thought: 'Someone wants to see me, *really* wants to see me.' My shoes hardly seemed to touch the pavement as Emma took me along to meet Don, and at the same time I thought, 'If it were not for Emma, none of this would be possible.'

Don had said he would pick us up at a point on the Mansfield Road, for a reason which brought the only cloud of the evening, and the only cloud surrounding our whole relationship. Don was still married and it was difficult to choose a time and place to meet. Friends had already told me that he and his wife no longer got on together, that the marriage did not work, and, in the way friends have of giving gratuitous advice, said I was foolish to become involved with a married man. Yet they had also told me that he was not the kind of man who would have casual affairs, so I knew that in order to ask me out, he must have thought seriously about the implications, and (this was a fond hope as much as a conclusion that I hardly dared think about) he must also have thought a great deal of me. For my part, I had no wish to encourage anyone to leave his wife. I felt strongly about this, and it was only because of what I learned about Don and the state of his marriage from my friends that my conscience was satisfied.

He took me that first evening to a little pub called The Three Wheatsheaves on the outskirts of Nottingham, near the university. I can remember few of the details, except it all seemed magical. The pub had a cosy, welcoming smell and atmosphere. Emma curled up under the table as we talked, and at one point Don tentatively took my hand. He was fifteen years older than me, and had this tremendous gift of making me, at twenty-one, feel I was the one person of importance in the entire universe. It seemed that we had been in the pub only a few minutes (although we must have been there for almost two hours) before I heard the landlord calling 'Time'. He had an extraordinarily deep voice, and sounded very jolly. In fact, whenever we went to his pub after that we never said, 'Let's go to the The Three Wheatsheaves.' We always called it The Gruff Man's Voice, and it became our private name for the very special place where we had our first evening together.

In the days that followed, I knew I was in love with Don. But did he love me? Somehow I thought it slightly unfair of me to expect such a thing, yet Don never gave a hint that my being unable to see was of any importance. His complete acceptance, in fact, provided my greatest encouragement to get on and be like everyone else, and to cover the frustrations of being blind. Therefore when someone said to me, 'It must be nice for you going out with Don. He must be a great help to you,' I used to become rather irritated. I hated the idea that a sighted person was a sort of spare limb to do things for me. Whatever else happened, I wanted to keep my independence.

But the doubts remained. The notion of a sighted person and particularly a handsome one, being in love with me was so far from what I had ever expected that it made me feel my whole world had been turned on its side. The logic seemed inescapable. Don could see. I was blind. Therefore he could not possibly be in love with me. At the same time I was certain, yet sceptical, of my own love for him. Love was something I had read about in braille paperbacks, and invariably concerned sighted people. How could it happen to me?

One evening Don rang me and said that the car had broken down, and he would not be able to meet me. I hardly heard him say, 'I've rung the garage, and they're coming along, and I'll ring you if they can put it right.' All I thought was: 'This is it. He's decided he doesn't want to see me any more. This is the excuse; he doesn't want to be involved with someone who's blind.'

'Yes,' I said, 'all right.' I put the phone down and paced up and down the flat, willing myself not to cry. Emma came up to me when at last I made some coffee and sat down. She rested her nose on my knee. We sat like that for hours. She understands, I thought.

The phone rang, and my heart turned over. It was Don again. 'I'm sorry, Sheila, they've had a look at it, and the alternator's gone; they can't get a new one till tomorrow. I *am* sorry ...' It was just as well that Anita happened to be away. I did not want to talk to anyone. I know I did not go to bed. I simply sat in a waking nightmare.

The next day I went about my work like an automaton, until just after ten o'clock I took an incoming call and heard the familiar voice. Don. As if nothing had happened, he said the car had been fixed, and what about meeting that evening instead? How could he have known what I had been through, or that my anxieties, rooted and fostered by my blindness, were all too quick to flourish? From then on I never doubted how much I loved Don. About a week later we were sitting in Don's car with the rain pouring down outside – somehow that made us feel more together. Don suddenly turned to me and said, 'It won't always be like this, you know.'

I didn't know what to say. I think I made some non-committal remark, yet knew the situation was changing, melting into something else.

Don went on, 'Will you wait till I'm free?'

I felt like opening the car door there and then, getting out and doing a dance with Emma on the pavement despite the pouring, freezing, December rain.

Would I wait? Of course I would!

7

Independence

So my life became centred around Don: snatching meetings whenever possible and experiencing a terrible emptiness whenever we were apart. At about this time I began to feel that my working life was in need of a change. Industrial Pumps had been taken over by another firm, and although I was perfectly able to carry on working there, the long journey back and forth to work was beginning to pall. It took Emma and me the best part of an hour. So when new management moved in, I decided to start looking for another job. If I had known then what frustration and misery this would entail, I suppose I might never have taken the decision. As it was it took me months to find somewhere else to work.

Before then I had never fully realised how terribly handicapped a blind man or woman is in the world, and the main difficulty, which began to become an obsession, was that others would not accept me. Don accepted me without question, so did Anita; yet their enlightened attitudes had possibly cushioned me against the indifference and outright rejection of so many of the rest of the human race.

I had nearly eight years' experience of working a busy switchboard and was as efficient as the next telephonist. But despite this, I was not good enough, apparently, for most employers. I used to take the *Nottingham Evening Post* home every night, and when Anita was back, she read down the 'Sits Vac' column for me, while I made a note in braille of the numbers. When I rang the firms concerned the dialogue went along these lines:

'I'm enquiring about the vacancy you've advertised for a telephonist.'

'Ah yes, could you give us some details of your experience?'

I would then tell them about my job, and how I was used to working a PABX Number Two type switchboard.

'Good, that sounds fine.'

Then I would drop the bombshell: 'There's something else I must tell you. I'm a blind person, but that doesn't make any difference to my ability to operate the switchboard, and I have a guide dog.'

I needn't have bothered. I could almost hear the waning of interest over the phone, like a balloon deflating.

'Ah yes, well thank you for calling. We'll keep you in mind, but we have had quite a few applicants already.'

This, at least, was some attempt to cushion the blow. But from time to time, the reception was brutally insensitive:

'Oh, I'm sorry, we couldn't possibly consider employing anyone who's blind. The office you'd have to work in is upstairs.'

'But my dog and I go up and down stairs every day of our lives.'

'I'm sorry, we couldn't possibly consider you. I'm afraid you'd be too much of a risk.'

When I tried to argue the point with the boss of one firm, he actually put the phone down on me.

Worst of all, perhaps, was the way that vacancies magically became filled as soon as I mentioned that I was blind. The utter dishonesty and hypocrisy made me want to scream. Eventually I decided that there was only one way round the problem. If I was to be considered ineligible just because I was blind, I simply would not mention the fact. I would give my qualifications and if asked to go for an interview, confront my prospective employers. It was desperation, but I had nothing to lose.

So that is what I did. As a result, I had two firms interested immediately, and both wanted to interview me on the same day. At the first firm I went to, some lace manufacturers, of which there are several in

Nottingham, dating from the days the Huguenots settled there, I sensed that they were surprised when I turned up with a guide dog. But Emma settled down at once and curled up beside me as I sat opposite the man asking the questions. Everything went off without a hitch. The office manager was then called in, and took me down to where the switchboard was. I felt it to see if it was the same type that I was used to, and it was. 'But,' he said, 'how do you operate it? It's not adapted for a blind person.' So I explained about the Post Office converting them free, and the job was offered to me on the spot.

It was a marvellous feeling to be able to go to the second interview knowing that whatever happened I would be taking a new job. The next vacancy was at Whytecliffe's, a big garage not far from the middle of Nottingham. Once again they were surprised at Emma, but having been presented on their doorstep with the prospect of a blind employee, they made no bones about going through the usual procedure. Emma again curled up quietly, this time under my chair. But although she just lay there, she played an important part in the interview. The Personnel Manager who asked me the questions was, it turned out, a breeder of Springer spaniels. His enquiries concerned Emma almost as much as my expertise with a switchboard, and I quickly formed the impression that he had become besotted at first sight with the chocolate-coloured creature under my chair. When I told him all the incredible things that Emma did for me, it was, I am sure, a deciding factor. I was offered the job, and I took it in preference to the other partly because the money was better, and also because Whytecliffe's was only a fifteen-minute walk from the flat.

I started as soon as I had worked out my notice at Industrial Pumps, during which time the Post Office engineers had been into Whytecliffe's and converted the switchboard – a praiseworthy service for which the Post Office should get full credit. The other girls in the office were surprised when I arrived on the first morning with a big Labrador. Most of them realised that Emma was a guide dog, but one girl came up to me and said, 'How is it you can bring your dog to work? It's not fair. I'd like to bring mine.' She was taken aback when I explained why Emma was there.

One or two of the girls began to doubt that I was really blind at all. They had looked out of the office windows and watched Emma and me coming down the street, crossing the zebra crossing, and coming straight to the door of the office, and could not believe that it was Emma who was responsible. In addition, Emma was so good at taking me anywhere I wanted to go inside the office, that I soon learned how to get about on my own. Despite the fact that they had seen me operating the switchboard by touch, taking messages in braille, and feeling my notebook for numbers, they began to think there was some catch. They thought that somehow – for what reason I was supposed to be doing it I have never fathomed – I was perpetrating an enormous hoax.

So they decided they would settle the matter. I worked at the top end of a long office that had desks on either side, and a narrow gangway in between. At the opposite end was the canteen. After Emma had taken me there for the first few days at tea break, I didn't bother to put on her harness for this little walk; I knew the direction and feel of the way well enough myself: straight down the passageway between the desks, turn right, through the door into the canteen. Emma came too, but she always raced well ahead of me, because she knew there would be a bowl of milk waiting for her in the canteen.

What happened on the morning the girls decided to find out about my blindness may sound mean, even cruel; it was certainly thoughtless, but I am sure it arose from quite genuine, though stupid, suspicions. What they did was to leave chairs and other objects in my way. So when the moment came for morning tea, Emma charged off in front of me, and I immediately crashed from obstacle to obstacle, finally knocking over and smashing a pair of steps. The silence after these had gone down, and I had let off steam, was a silence of deep embarrassment. One girl later came and said she was sorry, but they really did think I could see. My own reaction, once I had got over the whole business, was of even greater pride in Emma, that she could convince them that I was not blind at all.

Living as we did in Peel Street, and working at Whytecliffe's, Emma became very familiar with the centre of Nottingham. She learned the names of all the shops and bus stations I used. We did a lot of shopping at the big Co-op in Parliament Street. I only had to put her harness on, say 'Find the Co-op, Emma', and off we would go, her tail wagging furiously. She adored shopping. One of the reasons she liked it so much was because she made the rules. Rule One was that we could go shopping anywhere we liked, anywhere at all, but the first shop visited had to be a pet shop. Wherever we went, the route had to be planned to take in one of these vital stores. We would go in, buy bone-shaped biscuits, chews, vitamin chocolate drops or a rubber toy, and after that the rest of the operation could proceed. However, on the way to the Co-op we had to pass a second pet shop, although 'pass' is not strictly accurate. We would reach it, Emma would stop, and with her front paws on the step, imply: 'Well, here we are at another pet shop, just in case you've forgotten anything at the usual one.' I would say, 'No, no, come on Emma, find the Co-op.' And she was very good-natured in accepting that her suggestion had been turned down.

Rule Two about shopping was that we should never, whatever else was happening, and no matter how many of them lay along the route, miss an opportunity of visiting a butcher's shop. It was a terrible weakness of Emma's, and we became known in every butcher's within a five-mile radius of the middle of Nottingham. We would be going along, and I might, as well as concentrating on Emma, be thinking what Anita and I were going to have for supper, when suddenly, with no warning whatsoever, I would find myself in a shop with sawdust under my feet, and an unmistakable smell, and with no intention of buying so much as an ounce of mincemeat. Very embarrassing. But the butchers took it all in good part and got to know Emma so well that occasionally she got a bone for her initiative, and, of course, her good looks.

Yet once seriously down to the business of shopping, Emma was quite amazing. Her mind was an encyclopaedia of shop names. I would have only to say the word, and we were there. She was equally astonishing, if not more so, in a big store such as the Co-op. She knew not only how to get there but also the location of every department and every counter. I would have only to say, 'Find the Food Hall, Emma', or 'Find the Chemist' or 'Find the Shoe Department', and I would be taken there with never a mistake, and no hesitation, through the mill of other shoppers, and the various tempting smells.

She also knew what the words 'stairs' and 'lift' meant. She enjoyed using the lift in the Co-op, but did not much like the stairs. When I gave her the word to find the lift she made a vigorous dash, dragging me with her, in order to be first in, whether or not there was a crowd waiting. Occasionally I would want to go up only a single floor, so I would say, 'We won't wait for the lift, Emma, we'll go up the stairs. Find the stairs.' Find the stairs? At this word of command Emma would head immediately for the lift.

One evening in the spring of 1969 Anita came home and seemed very subdued. 'Sheila,' she said, 'I've got something to tell you: the office is going to move me to Grantham.'

'Oh,' I said. 'When?'

'Not until July,' she said, 'but I feel dreadful because I know you can't afford to keep the flat on by yourself.' This was true. I earned £9 a week at the time, and the rent we shared was £6 a week. The whole thing came as a shock, and it was sad to be suddenly presented with the prospect of breaking up our happy partnership.

Of course, what I longed to do more than anything else was to marry Don. But he still wanted to wait because he had a young daughter, Susan, and he felt he had a responsibility not to leave home until she was older and could understand what was happening. He felt we should wait until she was fourteen, and she wasn't ten yet. He was desperately afraid that Susan would not accept me, and would grow up blaming him for a breach in her family life. As it happened, I did not agree with him, but I respected his reasons. Yet the waiting was hard on both of us; it seemed like eternity.

There was a lot of waiting for Don, because he invariably did not finish at the surgery until about nine in the evening, and very often was kept even later by patients. Sometimes, if it had started to rain, Emma and I would be just about wet through by the time he arrived. Don once told me that it was seeing us both standing there waiting, and looking like orphans – me with my woolly hat soaked, and Emma's coat dark and her tail down – that made him realise how much I cared for him. He told me, 'I was drawing up by the kerb, and you hadn't heard the car because of the rain, and the pair of you looked a pitiful sight, it was terrible, and I thought, "That girl, she must love me".'

The prospect of living alone filled me with misgivings. It was of course the ultimate step towards genuine independence: but it also meant I really had to be able to fend for myself. I had no fears of being lonely, because Emma was there, and with her help I felt quite capable of coping. But there would be no one to read my letters for me, no one there to tell me the instructions on a packet of instant soup, or cake mix. What would I do if a fuse went? The light did not matter, but the iron or a power point did. On the plus side, I would be able to plan the flat so that I would know exactly where everything was: how the settee lay in relation to the table, and the table's position relative to the door, and no one would make even the slightest alteration to things as I had left them.

There was nothing for it but to set about looking for somewhere else to live, and at least there was a bit of time in which to do it. Luckily, I had been for some time on the local council housing list; I went to the housing officers, but there was nothing available. However, they were very pleasant, and noted my circumstances. The weeks ticked by. There was nothing I could afford in the local papers, or through the house agents, so I went to see the council again: with time running out I was getting desperate. This time they said they would do what they could as quickly as possible; but I think I probably owe the result more to Emma sitting in the office looking pathetic than to my own powers of persuasion: the man who interviewed me on this occasion made a great fuss of her, and she responded in her most appealing way. Within a week I had a letter offering me a flat in a block on the Ilkeston Road, about four miles from where we were living at the time.

I was greatly relieved; but then came the bad news. Animals were not allowed in the flats, and, though an exception could be made because Emma was a guide dog, I would have to part with Tiss. Rules apart, it would have been cruel to keep him in the block, but it did not make me any less downhearted. He and Emma had become very attached to each other. Tiss would always wait for us in the evening, sitting on the gate of the Peel Street house, and often spent the night sleeping on top of Emma. I wondered what the best course was, and then decided to put an advertisement in the *Nottingham Evening Post*. After a day or two there was a phone call from a family in Beeston. I questioned them very closely about their background because I was determined Tiss should go to a good home. They seemed the right sort of people, and we made an appointment for them to come along and see him. The strange thing was that on the day they were due to arrive, Tiss seemed to know what was afoot, and he disappeared. We finally found him in the attic. I heard from the family later that Tiss had settled down and seemed quite happy, but I could not bear to accept their invitation to go and visit him. He had been so much a part of our lives, and I think I should have been overcome at meeting him again in strange surroundings.

When the time came near for us to move out of Peel Street, there were cardboard boxes all over the place, and Emma knew what was going on. Far from being upset at the prospect of another move, she was determined not to be left out of what appeared to her to be an exciting game. Every time I started to pack a box, she would bring all her squeaky rubber toys and bones and so on, and drop them one by one into the box. That was constructive as far as it went. Unfortunately, as soon as I filled one box, and started on another, I would feel down into what should have been emptiness, and find that it too was being filled with squeaky toys, etc. So I had to go solemnly through the ritual of packing up all Emma's belongings, then unpacking them, and transferring them to the next box along the line. It was time-wasting, but Emma did not care. She stood by and approvingly wagged her tail.

When the new flat at last fell vacant, my mother came along to help clean it up. We got to the block of flats, and it seemed they were all the same, each one a little box on what I imagined to be a never-ending series of floors, all identical, and to which there was access by lift, or steps, or ramp. It was a gloomy experience, this first encounter with our new home. It took my mother ages to find Number 103, the flat we had been allotted, and when at last we got in and put our luggage and cleaning gear down, she said: 'Sheila, this is terrible. I'm so worried. You'll never find your way in and out of this block. Whatever possessed the council to give a blind person a flat on the fifth floor?'

'But, Mum,' I said, 'I've got Emma. I don't need a special place because I can't see. I just don't want that sort of thing.'

But she persisted. 'No, I'm going down to the council tomorrow to see about it, and get it changed.'

I pleaded with her. 'No, Mum, don't. I really don't want special treatment. It's perfectly all right. Emma's quite capable of taking me in and out.'

I finally persuaded her, and we got down to cleaning round the place and getting it ready for the furniture to arrive in a minivan which Bob, a friend of ours, was lending us. In the preceding weeks I had managed to round up, through the goodwill of all sorts of people, some furniture that would at least start me off after the furnished tenancy in Peel Street. My mother let me have a settee and a bed, friends had turned up trumps with tables and chairs and so on. Don gave me a table for the phone to stand on when it was eventually installed, and the only thing I had to buy was a gas cooker. When we had cleaned the flat more or less to my mother's satisfaction, we stopped for tea. But there were no provisions as yet, so one of us had to go out to the grocer's. My mother immediately said, 'I'll go.'

'No, no,' I said, 'I'll go with Emma. We'll make a start on getting to know the area.'

She was horrified, and it was evident that she was also still worried. 'No, Sheila,' she said, 'I'm not letting you go down there on your own.'

So, back to the old argument. 'But, Mum, I shan't *be* on my own. I've got Emma. We've got to start some time, it might just as well be now.'

I knew that Emma, in fact, was probably more capable than my mother and I put together, but I did not say so. At last, after further persuasion, she finally gave in. As Emma and I went down the hall, my parting words were, 'If we're not back in three days, call the RSPCA.'

To be fair, my mother had not seen Emma's skill at working in a new area, because she had brought me to the new flat, and Emma had had an off-duty spell. It might almost have been better, and quicker, if I had relied on Emma to begin with. Anyway, we set off along the open-sided landing. Emma had no difficulty in finding the lift, and we got out at the ground floor. But since I did not know the surroundings at all, I could not follow my usual procedure of asking Emma to find a particular shop. Instead, I had to ask her to find a shop, any shop, where I could ask for directions. I said to her as we went along, 'Emma, we're going to buy some tea, sugar and milk.' Whether by fluke, or because Emma actually recognised its appearance I shall never know, but the very first shop we tried was a corner grocery store. After we had bought the things we needed, we set off back: into the lift (I had to count the buttons to the fifth one up), along the passageway, and back without hesitation to the right door. My mother was amazed, and, in spite of the evidence, still found it difficult to accept Emma's ability.

I went out to ring Don. My mother had told me where she had seen a call box. It was just across the main road outside the flats. Emma knew the words 'phone box' and she took me straight across the road and to the kiosk I wanted. But when I got inside and felt for the receiver, it was missing. I ran my fingers down the wire, and this soon came to an end in my hand. The box had obviously been vandalised. I felt terribly frustrated and, worse, had no idea what to do. I was desperate to ring Don and tell him how the move had gone and what the new flat was like. I said to Emma, 'There's no phone, Emma. What are we going to do?'

I finally decided we had better search around, and hope that someone would come by who could tell us where another public telephone was. So I told Emma to take us along the road. But she did not respond. Instead she took me back across the main road, and I imagined she thought I had made my call and we were heading back to the flat. 'No, Emma,' I said, 'I haven't made my call. We've got to find another box. Come on let's go down this road.' So on we went, but she made no attempt to turn in where I judged the flats would be, and we carried on with me protesting. She then took me down a strange side road that had a rough feel to it underfoot, with bricks and bits of rubble (I learned later that both demolition and building were going on here at the same time). I tried to get Emma to stop, but she went on relentlessly, across the uneven ground until she turned left into another road and then sat down. I sensed that there was something there, put my hand out, and felt the ridged metal ribs and glass of a kiosk. 'Emma,' I said, 'how can you be so clever? How could you *know*?' She beat her tail on the pavement, but how she had managed to get us there has remained an unsolved mystery. Neither of us had ever been along that road before in our lives.

8

Evening Classes

THE EVENING CLASS that I had joined with Anita reflected our separate passions for writing and reading. My reading was done mainly with the help of talking books, a marvellous system of cassettes for the blind, recording a huge range of authors from Thomas Hardy to Ian Fleming.

Subsequently, however, a new suggestion came up. Kath Hill, another guide dog owner rang up one evening and said, 'Sheila, what do you think about beginning evening classes specially for the blind?'

My immediate reaction was, 'It sounds a marvellous idea. But what kind of classes?'

'Make-up and beauty,' she replied. 'I've had a call from someone who wants to start a class for blind people on this sort of thing, provided there's sufficient support. Do you think enough people would be interested?'

'Well,' I said, 'I most certainly would be. I'm sure lots of others would as well.'

We talked a bit more about the possibilities, and the more we discussed it, the more attractive the idea became. I had always worn some make-up, but had never been able to do anything elaborate. I used foundation cream and lipstick – foundation cream was easy to put on because it went all over the face, and lipstick, too, was quite simple because I was able to feel my lips and so not smear it. The prospect of other beauty aids was very appealing.

So the course was arranged by the Derbyshire Education Committee, and, in particular, by David Selby, who at the time was head of the Adult Education activities. He was a very forward-looking man, someone who thought beyond the confines of the subjects normally taught at evening classes, and he had a particular interest in catering for the blind.

The numbers had to be limited, of course, so that the teacher could cope. I rang round all my blind friends, and there was a good response. One of the major problems – how to get to Sandiacre, about ten miles away, just over the Derbyshire border – was being tackled in advance. An approach had been made to the Nottingham Blind Institution for a minibus to take us there.

The first evening brought great excitement. About ten of us had enrolled including six with guide dogs, and as we joined the minibus much greeting and tail-wagging went on, particularly between Emma and Kath's dog Rachel.

Our teacher was Joan Dickson and in spite of the fact that she had no experience with the blind, she was very encouraging. That first evening she dealt with basic skincare. She told each of us what skin type we had, and what colour hair; she explained which colour eyes usually went with which kind of hair, and how the foundation cream to be used was determined – for instance a peach foundation, medium tone, being required for brown hair and dark eyes like mine.

She also told us about face packs, something blind people would normally never think of using. But the best part of the course came later, when we had to use various kinds of make-up we had never before thought possible: eyeshadow, mascara and eyeliner. I had no idea how to apply them. Joan started by telling us, 'First of all, you have to match your colours. If you're going to wear a green dress, then you want a green eyeshadow.' It may sound odd, but that had never occurred to me, and it was a minor revelation. 'Then,' she went on, 'you have to match your lipstick to your eyeshadow and dress, and, in the case of a green dress and eyeshadow you could use a pink shade of lipstick.' I was fascinated.

But the problem still remained: how actually to apply the eyeshadow? Joan came round to each one of us and demonstrated, and by feeling we learned. She put the eyeshadow on me, and I realised it could be done by touch, and that the bone above the eye and at the side is a good guide, while the eyelash could be felt as a limiting landmark for shadow. Mascara was a little more difficult, and even with practice we only partially succeeded. No one found it possible to put mascara on the lower lashes. Eyeliner was easier because the line of the top of the lashes could be felt and followed. But although I say it was easier, it all took a lot of practice and a lot of care before we got it right, and Joan was endlessly patient in coming round and telling us how we were getting on. Fairly frequently we had to take off whatever we had put on and start all over again.

Nail varnish was another beauty aid Joan dealt with. Up to then, I had used nail varnish, but by the technique of covering my nails and the surrounding skin. When it was dry, I would peel off the varnish from the skin. A girl at work had once watched me doing this, and observed: 'You're getting varnish all over the skin round your nails. I'd always thought how beautifully you put it on.' I replied, 'Well, now you know how I do it.' But Joan helped me to apply the varnish correctly and efficiently by touching the outside of the nail first, over the cuticle, then brushing upwards to the top.

The class was a huge success, and it made me feel marvellous when I was going out with Don because at last I could make myself up properly. People we met sometimes asked, 'Who put your make-up on for you?' I was now able to answer, 'I did,' and it gave me a terrific feeling of completeness, and of being equal to everyone else.

The make-up and beauty classes in fact went so well, and David Selby was so impressed by the results, that it was decided to hold further evening classes solely for the blind. The next session, we tackled flower arrangement. Colours, of course, were an obvious obstacle. Yet some flowers, with so many differing leaves and petal shapes, can be learned by touch, and hence the colours can be learned too. As daffodils are unmistakable to the fingers, it can be known immediately that there is a yellow flower. Similarly, chrysanthemums are easy to identify, and so bronze or deep red or yellow is the scheme for the arrangement.

In addition, what we had learned in the make-up and beauty class about matching colours was useful here. People had told me that various colours matched, or clashed violently, but it was not until doing these evening classes that I really fixed the various possible and impossible combinations in my mind. Applying all this knowledge, and using the pin-holders we were taught about, we came up with some quite respectable displays.

The next course, dressmaking, was an even bigger adventure. There had been dressmaking classes at my school, but I had never been allowed near the sewing machine, and such attempts as I had made unfailingly turned out badly. The teachers at school had no technique for teaching a blind pupil something for which sight seemed an indispensable asset. But the evening classes under our two teachers, Irene and Hazel, were very different.

We started with basic techniques. We were all given small pieces of material, and shown how to tack by making loops, using wool, or stronger thread, instead of ordinary fine cotton so we could know what we were doing by touch. Then we were given skirt patterns. But instead of the ordinary kind of tissue patterns that are bought in shops, these were made of much thicker paper, almost the texture of wallpaper. Hazel and Irene had given this great thought and decided that with a stiffer paper we would be able to cut out the patterns ourselves. They had made dots about an inch from the edge all round, so that once we had cut out the patterns, they could be folded back and we could feel these dots in order to do the tacking. They had cut holes in the pattern where the darts were meant to be, so that we tacked round the darts while we still had the pattern on the piece of material, and when we took it off, we could feel where we had tacked. This was a marvellous innovation for the blind, and Hazel and Irene had achieved it by themselves wearing blindfolds and, by trial and error, discovering what a blind person might or might not be able to accomplish.

Next came work on the electric sewing machine. On all the controls of the machine there were braille instructions, and Hazel and Irene had also had a needle guard fitted, as well as a guide – in the shape of a long metal strip – to ensure that we put the material through straight.

Yet much as I admired all this, and felt I would be able to handle the machine properly, I was rather reluctant to make my first attempt. I heard everyone else using the machine, and it whirred away busily. Then Hazel came over and said, 'Come on, your turn Sheila.' 'Is it?' I said. 'Surely there's someone else before me.' 'No,' said Hazel, 'everyone else has been. Come on, it won't bite you.'

I went over to the machine and felt it gingerly all over, and said, 'What if I get my hand under the needle and stitch my fingers?' 'You won't,' said Hazel, 'there's a needle guard.'

So I had to start, and once I had got my piece of material in the machine all went reasonably well. I found I had to be careful about the speed, which was controlled by a foot pedal. I chose a slow speed so I could feel what I was doing in time to avoid mistakes. At first I could feel the material slipping through my fingers and didn't know what was happening to it. So I went a little crooked on the sewing but Hazel was beside me to help, and eventually I mastered the technique, although that still didn't prevent me from making some blunders that would have instantly earned me the sack in a commercial rag trade establishment.

I was making, for instance, a pair of trousers, and was left to machine them up myself. But when I felt the result of all my work I could not understand what had happened. Instead of a pair of trousers I had produced a very long skirt! I had sewn all the wrong seams together. On another occasion, I produced a dress with one sleeve inside, and one outside. Nevertheless, if I knew I would never work for Hardy Amies, I still had a marvellous time, as did everyone else in the class. Some of them had far more ability than I, and made really pretty clothes, and while – despite aids such as braille tape measures – we all needed some sighted help for dressmaking (Don used to come to the rescue when taking up hems and getting measurements right), we all felt, when the course was over, we had achieved something really valuable for ourselves.

I suppose that the great thing about the evening classes was that they widened our confidence in our own capabilities. So much so that several of us got together and decided we should like to start a drama group for the blind in Nottingham. We knew there were similar groups in other places. In London, for example, there was one at the Jewish Blind Centre. So we went ahead. We obtained permission from our own local Blind Institution to hold rehearsals on their premises and found two drama teachers to help us.

At the first meeting, several problems presented themselves. We chose two short one-act plays: *Companion to a Lady* by Stanley Houghton, and *The Dear Departed* by Mabel Constanduros and Howard Agg, but we had to decide how we were going to learn our parts. One of the teachers suggested that a recording could be made of the plays, and so we would be able to learn our lines from tape. This was fine; the next task was to work out how we were going to get about the stage. Fairly obviously we could not take our dogs with us. In the end it was decided that the stage would be exactly measured out for us, as well as the distances between each prop and piece of furniture, and a strip of carpet would be put at the front of the stage just before the footlights, to prevent us striding off the stage into Row A. This worked, though it meant that in addition to learning the lines, we had to learn each movement, whether it was seven paces upstage and turn to the right, five paces from the wings and face outwards, or two paces to the left and exit stage right.

We had great fun at rehearsals until, at last, the night of our first dress rehearsal arrived. It was the night before the actual show. We had been booked for two nights at a local amateur theatre, and all the tickets had been sold out. I had to run on to the stage because someone had attempted to murder my aunt, rush forward, reach the carpet-strip (and so know I was next to the bed my aunt was sitting on), sit down beside her and put my arm round her to comfort her, then go over to the telephone in the left-hand corner of the stage and dial the police. During rehearsals we had no telephone, and simply pretended there was one. By the time of the dress rehearsal most of the props were in place, but I had been told a few days before that there would not be an actual telephone until the first night.

Unfortunately, things did not go as smoothly as we had hoped. My piece, in fact, was a disaster from beginning to end. I whisked on to the stage, shouting 'Aunty, I'm here, I'm here', and dashed over to her. I felt the carpet-strip, turned round to sit on the bed, missed it completely, dragged her on to the stage with me, and we both sat in a heap, dying with laughter. To my horror, I heard more laughter – from out front – and it was only then that I realised an audience had been invited to watch the dress rehearsal. I was so embarrassed. When I had recovered and dusted myself down, I rushed over to where the phone was meant to be, pretended to pick it up and dial the police, and then made my exit to some rather puzzling murmurings from the audience.

I walked straight into the arms of the director

backstage, and she immediately hissed at me, 'What were you playing at? What about the phone, then?'

'Well, I did that bit, I did that bit,' I said.

'No, the phone was there,' she said, 'you fool. You were about an inch away from it, pretending to pick it up, and it was there all the time. The audience couldn't make out what you were playing at.'

But that was not the end of the evening's misfortunes. We all went on to take a curtain call, and the girl who had played my aunt had lost one of her slippers. When we were all on stage, she said, 'Quick. I've lost one of my slippers, help me find it.' So when the curtain went up, there we were, on our hands and knees. I suppose stranger things have happened in the history of British drama but I cannot imagine what they might be.

It was about this time in my life that I became an Avon representative. One evening Don and I were discussing my finances (never very healthy) and I asked him if he thought there was anything I could do to earn a little over and above my wages from my daily job at the garage. I was well aware that not being able to see narrowed the field of opportunities, but I thought there must be something I could do. As it happened, an Avon representative had called on Don that evening, and he suggested I could do that.

At first thought, I was dubious. 'Oh, Don,' I said, 'I really couldn't go round to people's houses and flats trying to sell them things, and there's a lot of form-filling entailed, you know, which I couldn't do.'

'Yes, you could,' said Don, 'and if there was much form-filling, I could do it for you. Why don't you ring them up and get one of their area representatives to call?'

In the end I was persuaded, particularly since I could take a small tape recorder round with me and talk all the sales details into the microphone. I rang up the local Avon representative and she came round to tell me all about their selling scheme, and how to process the orders, and so I was in business. I decided that I would limit myself, to begin with at least, to the three hundred flats in my block and the adjoining ones; I knew how to get round them without much difficulty. So we set off. Emma, I think, did not know what to make of it, since we stopped at every door and knocked. But things worked out well. The numbers on the doors were raised and I could feel where I was, and if people happened to be out when I knocked, I simply recorded their number on tape so I could call again the following evening.

The response was far better than I could have thought possible. I found a lot of people interested in the beauty products I was selling, and, very often, I was invited in for a cup of tea. But my success was due in no small part to Emma. Most of the people in the flats had seen her out with me, and, apart from being interested in the Avon scheme, they also welcomed the opportunity to say hello to Emma. Quite possibly she sat in mute appeal: 'Please buy something, or she won't be able to feed me tomorrow.' Whether or not this was the case, I have no idea, but the orders came in very well. About once a week we would translate them off the tape, and Don would spend hours filling the forms in.

It was a rewarding extension to my life, and not only financially. Through the scheme I got to know a whole new circle of friends. In addition, I used to meet people who quite obviously rarely went out except to do the shopping, and hardly had anyone to visit them. There were a lot of lonely people in those flats, and I think they liked me calling, and seeing someone they could talk to. It was astonishing, too, how I found myself able to help in other ways. Because I had done the make-up and beauty class, I was able to give advice. A surprising number of women used to want guidance about what kind of shades they should wear. I used to ask, 'What colour hair have you got? What colour eyes? What sort of tone would you say your skin is?' And as a result I would say what shades I thought best.

This really was marvellous, and gave me great confidence. I thought: 'Here I am blind, but I can help these people.' I hope not too many of them went around with the wrong colour lipstick as a result!

9

Emma Saves My Life

AFTER EMMA AND I had been together for about a year, I decided I should like to become an official speaker on behalf of Guide Dogs: to go round and tell people about their work, and help raise funds. Emma had given me so much, I wanted to try and help. Not only that, I was anxious for the opportunity to tell people how marvellous she was, and all about her.

The first talk I ever did came about through Anita. She invited me to one of her church meetings. She said she had told everyone in her circle so much about Emma that they were all dying to meet her. Off we went, and I felt on top of the world; this was what I wanted to do. We got to the hall, Anita met us, and we sat in one of the back rows. I could sense that there were a lot of people (about one hundred and fifty I was told later). They started with hymns and prayers, and in the middle of 'Lead Us, Heavenly Father, Lead Us' I suddenly realised I was scared stiff. I thought: 'What on earth persuaded me to do this sort of thing? I'm going to have to stand up in front of all these people, and *talk*. I must be mad.' When the hymn came to an end, there was a terrible, expectant silence. I heard someone announcing that they had a speaker. Even worse, I then, with a thump in my heart, heard my name.

They asked me if I would go to the front. I put Emma's harness on, took hold of the handle, and told her to go forward. Up the aisle she went, and took me onto the platform. I had hoped for moral support from her; but it was fairly clear that none would be forth-coming. As soon as she turned and, obviously, caught sight of the audience, Emma went round behind me, curled up, and put her nose through my feet in an atti-tude that plainly indicated: 'You carry on doing whatever you have to; I'm well hidden.'

I spoke, I suppose, for about five minutes. It seemed like five hours. I stuttered and stammered through what had happened at the training centre, and tried to put over what Emma meant to me. The sole compensation was that, unlike sighted speakers, I could not be distracted by the faces in front of me. At the same time, I had no means, as I hesitated, faltered and blundered on with many an 'Er', and 'Well', of gauging their reac-tions. When I finally ran out of things to say – which did not take long – I just stood trembling, and to my amaze-ment there was a great burst of applause.

I could hardly believe it. Emma immediately leaped up from behind me, wagging her tail furiously (after all, the applause was for *her)*. Then she took her harness, which was on the floor by my feet, and rushed away down the hall. She went from row to row to show how clever she was, and of course everyone was delighted. From that moment Emma was certainly never shy of going to talks; as soon as I told her what we were about to do, there was no holding her back, she would go at double her usual rate.

All this meant a lot of hard work keeping records, but here Don came in again. I bought large diaries, and he kept them up-to-date, and we reviewed each week the forward plans. On Sunday afternoons we would get the diary out, Don would tell me all the information I wanted, then I would translate it through my braille machine, and carry the separate braille instructions for the week round with me to the various talks.

Only one thing ever deterred Emma from wanting to go on a talk, and that was rain. She did not like going out anyway when it was raining, and this made life a little difficult. I would have to drag her out, saying, 'Come on, you won't get wet. You won't feel it with your great, furry coat.' But Emma was aware, no doubt, that even if her coat protected her, she still had four big paws to slide about in the mud. Going to work, or more accurately, trying to persuade her to get me to work when it was raining, was a great performance. She would dig her paws in, and refuse to move outside the flats. I would beg, plead, cajole, and even threaten her (in the politest possible way). Eventually she would reluctantly move off, but I was often late, and I could never bring myself to tell the boss, 'It was Emma's fault.'

When I started giving talks I was struck by the odd questions people used to ask at the end. For instance, 'How do you find your clothes in the morning?' That stumped me. It was something I had never really thought about. What could I say, but, 'Normally in a heap on the chair where I left them.' I knew what they were getting at, but something that sighted people might imagine an immense difficulty or inconvenience is really not as complicated as all that when you are blind. You *know* where things are; it's your life.

The one thing I disliked about giving talks was the dinner that sometimes preceded the actual lecture. I remember one particularly dreadful occasion when I had to tackle a fruit cocktail. It contained pineapple chunks. Some idea may be gained of the problem by putting on a blindfold and attempting to chase pineapple chunks round a dish with a spoon. Very elusive they are. I stuck to it, knowing by the lack of eating sounds around me that everyone was watching, and feeling the tension rising. It happened to be a warm summer evening, and I had on a rather low-cut dress. I finally captured a chunk and raised it in my spoon, when I suddenly became aware that it was attached to several other chunks in a kind of string. Worse, the shock of this made me drop the spoon – and the entire string of pineapple disappeared down my cleavage. Not the best start to an evening!

Well-meaning 'help' was constantly being offered, particularly on my arrival. I would be given a seat and told 'Now, don't move.' I always think it strange that so many people regard the blind as rather dangerous and unstable explosive material, which, if allowed the least chance of independent life and movement, may cause some sort of cosmic disaster. Quite apart from that, the blind are often treated as deaf as well, if not mentally defective. The admonition, 'Don't move', was frequently a sort of military command: 'DON'T MOVE!' I would sit there, tense and afraid lest someone else suddenly grabbed me and forcibly propelled me elsewhere. I would take Emma's harness off, and then start to take my coat off. That was always fatal. The instant I stood up to do so, I was pounced on from all sides: 'What do you want? What is it? Why are you *moving*?'

The thing that spurred me on through all these minor tortures was knowing that when I stood up to speak, *they* would be the ones who could not move, and I would be able to demonstrate to them that I was just like any other human being apart from not being able to see. When I stood up at the beginning, I could practically feel the tension generated at the thought of listening to someone who was blind: the last thing they wanted to do was to laugh. But somehow I succeeded in getting them to do just that, though it often took a little time.

Another of the rewarding results of my talks with Emma was that very often the organisations we visited decided not only to give a donation to the Association, but to try and raise the money to buy a guide dog. The full cost of a guide dog is £500, including the puppy-walking, the training of the dog at the centre, and the training of the blind person with the dog. The cost just of training the dog at the centre is reckoned at about £250. When a blind person goes for his or her dog they are not, of course, required to pay this sort of money (if they were I should either have had to rob a bank, or would still be sitting at home saving up). All that is asked is 50p and this enables blind people to have a dog no matter what their financial circumstances, and yet not to feel that they are accepting charity. It also means that a lot of effort goes into raising money for guide dogs, with many willing people all over the country devoting time and energy to it. So when my audience came up with the idea that they would like to contribute by provision of a guide dog, I was always delighted.

I once planned a fundraising event myself. I decided to do a twenty-mile sponsored walk (with Emma in the lead, of course). Don and I took a long time to plan this walk. We went from the flat in the car, and put it together bit by bit. Then we had to plan exactly how I was going to attempt it. In this we were lucky. Nottingham University has a department that deals with blind mobility, and the late Dr Alfred Leonard had come up with the idea that very small pocket tape recorders could be used for giving a blind person a route, say, from a map.

The route would be recorded, and the blind man or woman would take the tape recorder with them, listening in as they went. We arranged to borrow one of these little tape recorders from the university (they had only just come on to the market and were expensive) and Don and I got down to putting my route on tape.

Don came out with me, walking every yard of the way, and recording how many kerbs to cross, where to turn left or right, what sort of pavement would be under my feet, what sort of objects I would hear as I passed them, when I would pass through busy shopping areas, and when I would be in the country and going across fields. Don was marvellous at putting the right information on to the tape. Not 'then you turn left by the Post Office', but the more accurate information that I needed. He had an incredible instinct for it, but he did have his reservations about the walk.

'I don't know,' he said, after one of our route information sessions, 'it's a long way for you to walk, twenty miles.'

'Don't worry,' I said, 'I've got Emma.'

'Well yes, I know, but I don't like the idea of you going out there all on your own – both of you. What if you get lost?'

The route lay from Nottingham to Wollaton, Stapleford, Nuthall and back down the Alfreton Road to the flat. He had a point, even though I had Emma, and even though I said, 'I can always ask the way, I've got a tongue in my head.'

'I know. But I still don't altogether like the idea.'

The point was that I did not want him to come with me on the actual day, because this would rob the whole idea of its worth. But eventually we compromised. Don said, 'Well, I'll tell you what. We'll arrange checkpoints, and I'll meet you at various stages along the route.'

So that was fine. I had, in the event, the company of another guide dog owner, a friend of mine called Wendy who wanted to come along as well with her dog Candy. But Don, it was reassuring to think, would be in the background to make sure that nothing went wrong. We had chosen a Sunday for the walk, and it turned out to be a glorious morning. I got out my pocket tape recorder, and the four of us set off.

We had arranged the route on the Nottingham side to go via various parks, so that Emma and Candy could have as much free running as possible. We had agreed that if the dogs became too tired we would give up immediately. After all, it would not matter so much if we were on our last legs, but, in fairness, we had to think of the dogs because they would really be doing the hard work.

Both Wendy and I had haversacks, with packed sandwiches, bowls and a generous water supply, as well as something to eat for the dogs. Everything went well. In no time at all, it seemed, we were past the outskirts of Nottingham, and into the country on the Derbyshire side. Don turned up at the appointed checkpoints and made sure we were all right, and sent us on our way with appropriate encouragement. Well into the afternoon we were still going quite strong. I clicked the tape recorder on to get the next part of the route, and said to Wendy, 'Now, we've got to go under a bridge, so listen for a bridge. Immediately we've gone under it, we turn right, and we're on the main road back into Nottingham.'

'OK,' said Wendy, and we carried on. We seemed to have gone a long way, but no bridge turned up, and then, both dogs stopped.

'Did you hear us go under a bridge?' I asked.

'No, I haven't heard one.'

'Well, there's no point in us both getting lost. You stay here, and I'll investigate.'

I told Emma to go. She seemed rather reluctant. But eventually I managed to get her across the road we were on, and when I reached the other side I could feel gravel and loose stones under my feet instead of the pavement there should have been.

'This is peculiar, Emma. I wonder where we're going?' And she stopped again. I said, 'No, come on. This may be the continuation of the road. We're in the country. Perhaps the main road is down here some-where.' I tried to encourage her, and she went on, but very cautiously. Then I felt grass under my feet. At the same instant Emma stopped and refused to budge. I felt someone's breath on my neck, and was immediately struck with terror. I froze. I could not have moved for a fortune. Then my ear was shattered by a thundering 'Moo …' We were in a field full of cows. Or was it a bull? Who knows? We did not stop to find out. Emma and I were out of the field and back to Wendy and Candy in ten seconds flat.

When we retraced our steps – which we should have done before – we found the bridge, and were back on the right road.

The dogs never showed any signs of tiredness. When we got back they seemed good for another twenty miles. Wendy and I, on the other hand, staggered in exhausted.

But it was worth it. Sponsors paid up and we raised nearly £250.

Not long after this, Emma and I were asked to speak one evening in Newark, which is almost sixteen miles from Nottingham. It was a winter evening (the winter was the busiest time for talks, because the majority of organisations seemed to close down in summer, or arrange outings instead of speakers).

When Emma and I got off the bus at seven o'clock in Newark, there was no one to meet us. The place at which I was giving the talk was some way from the bus station, and I was expecting someone with transport to take us. It was very cold. Emma and I walked up and down. I felt my braille watch from time to time. Half-past seven came, but no one arrived. Then I thought: 'Have I made a mistake? Did I say the eight o'clock bus?' So we walked around a bit more. The eight o'clock bus duly rumbled in from Nottingham, but still no one arrived to pick us up. By this time I was not only cold, but very hungry as well. Something had obviously gone wrong, and at this point I was overcome by hunger. 'Emma,' I said, 'we're going for fish and chips. Can you find the scent?' So off we went, although I had never been to Newark before. Emma seemed much perked up by the prospect. We took a long time, endlessly searching the streets around the bus station, until, at last, I could smell the unmistakable and extremely alluring odour of fish and chips. Whether Emma had led me to it, or whether we found it by accident, I have no idea. But she had a reward anyway, and shared the bag of plaice and chips with me. Then we trailed back to the bus station, and a weary hour later were back in Nottingham.

I could not imagine what had gone wrong. It had been an utter waste of time. Even worse, I'd come away with no donation to the guide dogs.

We had been indoors only a few minutes before the phone rang. A voice said, 'Hello, this is Mansfield Young Wives here.'

'Oh, yes.'

'Where were you?'

'Where was I? When?'

'Tonight.'

Then it dawned. At the time we had been stamping the pavements of Newark bus station, there had been an impatient gathering of ladies stamping their feet in a hall in Mansfield. Oh dear. I suppose it was bound to happen sooner or later, but I could not apologise enough. What had happened, as it transpired when I checked with Don, was that he had quite firmly written 'Mansfield Young Wives' in the book. But, by some aberration, I had transcribed Mansfield into braille as Newark!

Generally I liked talking to WIs, Rotary Clubs and Round Tables – at the last of these Emma and I revelled in being the only females – but another sort of talk I always enjoyed immensely was a Cub or a Brownie meeting. Compared to adults, I found children so straightforward, unembarrassed and refreshing. Their questions were always imaginative, and they accepted me without question or reservation. I would never feel they were thinking, 'Poor thing, she can't see.' They took that for granted, and, in any case, were more fascinated by Emma and what she could do. Typically, the thing they were most interested in was the way that Emma worked with me. They wanted a demonstration. But this created a difficulty. When I became an official speaker for the Guide Dog Association it was stressed that on no account should demonstrations of this sort be given. The reasons are easy to understand: the dogs would be surrounded by people, surrounded by all sorts of distractions; they would be working in artificial conditions, which would not be fair on them. This was fine as a theory. But Emma never appreciated it, and seemed perfectly happy at a chance to show off. In fact, it would have taken someone with a stronger will than mine to deter her.

So I found the best way of satisfying children's curiosity was a simple little act. From where I stood at the far end of the hall I would say, 'I'm going to ask Emma to take me to the door, down the centre aisle. But if you'd like to put some obstacles in my path, then you'll see how Emma does her job and takes me round them.'

Emma was always delighted when this moment arrived. She thought it the most marvellous opportunity to display her intelligence. Children would strew the centre aisle to the door with coats and other paraphernalia, and occasionally the odd chair. Emma was pleased to outwit their every move. If she could not find a clear path down the middle, she promptly took me another way, round the side, to immense applause.

On one particular evening with the Cubs, however, things took a slightly different turn. We completed the talk, Emma had done her demonstration, and then I asked for questions. One very bright spark who sounded about seven was the first to stand up, and asked, 'Will Emma do anything anybody else tells her?'

'No, of course not,' I said, totally unaware of what he was planning, after listening carefully to my talk about some of Emma's likes and dislikes.

'If I call her to come to me, won't she come?'

'No, I'm afraid she won't.'

'Can I try?'

'Of course,' I said confidently, 'of course. Have a try.'

'Emma, Emma,' he shouted. Emma remained at my side, and I imagine I probably had a silly grin on my face. Then he tried something different. He shouted at the top of his voice:

'Emma, come on – butcher's ...' And Emma moved so fast, she was down the hall in two seconds.

Although I liked talking to children, I was rather dubious when an invitation to speak came from Woods School. This is an establishment for disabled children just outside Nottingham. When I spoke to the headmistress, she explained that many of the children were confined to wheelchairs, with diseases such as multiple and disseminated sclerosis, and spina bifida. All the children were to a greater or lesser degree crippled in their limbs and bodies. Some of them, apparently, had motorised carriages because their degree of paralysis was such that they were only just about capable of pressing the button to operate their wheels.

The headmistress asked me if I would go and talk to them, because the children would love to see Emma, and would like to know how a blind person coped with life. I was apprehensive. I felt, I suppose, as a sighted person does at the prospect of being confronted with someone who is blind. But I thought, I must go, and we made a booking.

When Emma and I arrived, I asked the headmistress 'Won't it be difficult to explain blindness? Their disabilities seem much greater than mine. Will it mean anything to them?'

To my surprise she said, 'We've talked about blindness in the classroom, and the children don't understand how you can get about when you can't see. They think it would be much worse to be blind than paralysed.'

I felt very strange, and could hardly agree. However, she suggested that we should speak to the younger children first. I got into the classroom, and then heard them coming in with their wheelchairs, and the sound of the buzzers that operated the electric ones. They were all very quiet as I told them about Emma. She, I think, was rather puzzled about the wheelchairs. As a result, she was more subdued than usual during the talk. I was fascinated by the children's questions. They were very intelligent. As I have said, most children I talk to don't really think about anyone not being able to see. They simply accept the fact. But these children, with their own handicaps, were far more aware. When I got to the older children, they were even more receptive and understanding, and as I talked to them, I found it heartbreaking knowing that some of them would not live very long. Yet I could not mistake their incredible zest and enthusiasm for life as they came up to take a closer look at Emma and make a fuss of her.

Two of them approached me and said, 'You must come to our swimming pool.' I had no idea there would be a swimming pool, but these boys explained that it was used for therapy. Some children, who were not mobile on land, were able to move in water.

One of the little boys was in a wheelchair and the

other was on crutches. I could hear the crutches going down the corridor as they led me to the swimming pool area. Then I heard the crutches go faster and faster, and it was becoming difficult for Emma, me and the boy in the wheelchair to keep up. It suddenly struck me that they were having a race! A race! I could hear the sound of the crutches becoming slightly more distant and the wheelchair speeding up. Then I was horrified to hear the little boy on crutches, whose name was Robin, fall with a terrible echoing crash of scattering metal sticks. I caught up with him, and had no idea what to do. Meanwhile, I could not understand why Philip, the boy in the wheelchair, was laughing his head off! Robin was on the ground and making the most strange noises. I knelt down beside him and asked, 'Are you all right?' There was no reply beyond these worrying noises. And then I realised that he, too, was helpless with laughter. It was infectious, and when I'd got him back on his crutches, we all set off again down the corridor, unable to stop laughing. What Emma made of it, I have no idea.

We got to the swimming pool, and I was fascinated to hear the children describe the little canoes in which they propelled themselves. There was a marvellous atmosphere, and we all got along well. I was able to ask them what it was like to be in a wheelchair, and all but one said something of the order, 'Well, it's quite normal, we don't think anything about it at all ... we can do this ... we can do that, and we can see, we can see to read, and see to play games, and ...' They felt sorry for me because I could not see. It was very humbling.

Another centre for the disabled I visited was Clifton Spinney, which is a rehabilitation centre for blind people not far from Nottingham. It is a residential place where people who have recently lost their sight can go for a month- or two-month course to help them re-shape their lives without the aid of sight. Because of the gradual way I had lost what little sight I ever had, I always considered myself fortunate compared with people who had enjoyed perfect vision and then lost it. Naturally I had the frustrations of being blind, but I had never at any point sat down and thought: 'Last year I could see, and now I can't; I shall never get used to this. What am I going to do?'

I always found it difficult if I met someone who had newly lost his or her sight. It is the worst way to go blind. People are such visual animals that sight over-rides every other sense. To have that sense suddenly taken away is a terrible blow. It brings with it not only physical blindness, but a kind of equivalent mental blindness as well. Sea anemones immediately close up when anything touches them. People who go blind seem to close up mentally in the same way. But they often remain shut off from the world.

So, if I had been dubious to begin with about going to talk to disabled children, I was doubly worried about the idea of talking to the blind at Clifton Spinney. The point was that one of the main aspects of the talks I gave was to prove to sighted people how normal blind people were, how they were able to cope and get on with their daily lives, and to put over how I had done it, and how Emma helped me. How could I say this to these people?

The Spinney was managed by a Mr and Mrs Spencer. Mrs Spencer was sighted, but her husband was blind. It was good that a blind person was in charge of the centre, because no one knows better what the blind require than someone who cannot see. Mrs Spencer was very kind. She picked me up and took me to the centre, and, once there, led me along to the room where I was to give the talk, and where a blind audience was already waiting. She left me saying that her husband would be along shortly to introduce me. I heard the door close. I sat on a little platform with Emma by me, and I realised that not only could I not see them, but they could not see me. The thought struck me forcibly, and I did not like it one bit. I wasn't used to mixing with blind people. I had always chosen the company of sighted people, and if I had blind people as friends it was always because I liked them personally, not because of, or with any allowance for, their not being able to see.

So I sat there, becoming more and more apprehensive, and my throat going drier and drier as I waited for Mr Spencer. I could hear the audience chatting among themselves, and noticed, not for the first time, that with the totally blind, particularly those who have been recently blinded, there is a characteristic and very monotonous tone to their voices, somehow reflecting the idea that in losing their sight, all hope and interest in life has gone as well. Then I heard Mr Spencer come through the door. 'Hello, Sheila, my name's Charles Spencer.' I stood up and moved towards his voice and put out my hand to shake his. We collided. My hand was somewhere on his jacket pocket, his was near my left ear. I felt flustered and disheartened, and thought: 'This is what happens when you put blind people together.'

I started off in the way I would begin one of my usual talks. But within a few minutes I knew I would have to change my tactics. I was getting no response whatever from the audience. There were no laughs at all, let alone in the right places. It was a terrible feeling, like talking into a vacuum. I had to get through to them somehow and eventually I did. But it was very hard work – I think the most difficult talk I have ever done.

Question time was correspondingly drastic: there was no sequence of questions, with one person asking after the other. Everyone shouted, and at times there were three questions in the air at the same time, and I could not understand one of them. This was not because newly blinded people are stupid, or have no feeling for other people, it is because they feel cut off, they have suddenly been thrust on this dark island, and they have to do their best to get away from it. Many of them were still suffering the shock of losing their sight, of having to begin a completely different life, of having their main sense taken from them.

I felt desperately sympathetic. One of the difficulties that affect the newly blind is that sighted people tend to make a fuss, and to encourage the feeling that, suddenly, they have become helpless, bereft almost of any faculties. They tend to take over, and do things for blind people which if they were taught they could do for themselves. So much is done that sometimes the blind person becomes convinced she or he really is incapable. One of the objects at Clifton Spinney was to counter this very real threat.

As the questions sorted themselves out, it became evident that they were particularly interested in guide dogs, so Emma played her part in convincing them that, despite blindness, they could have real mobility and freedom.

All the same I was truly glad to leave Clifton Spinney: this may seem a terrible thing to admit, but it's true. How thankful I was to have Emma, and for the start I had had in life. I could never have worked there as Mr

Spencer did. It would have been too close to home, too real. The problems at Clifton Spinney were all out in the open, and being tackled. But in their heart of hearts no blind person wants to admit that there is a problem in not being able to see.

How thankful I had to be for Emma was brought home to me some weeks after this. Going through town one day, she took me to a zebra crossing at a busy point. I heard a bus or a lorry pull up to let us cross. I gave Emma the signal to go forward, and we started to go over the crossing. But we had taken only a step or two before Emma stopped, and began to back away, tugging on the harness. I could not understand what she was doing, and entirely forgot to trust her. 'Emma, come on, it's all right, they've stopped for us,' I urged. She would not move, however, and I thought I must step out to show that everything was clear – because I could hear the engine of the bus or lorry safely ticking over and waiting for us. So I stepped forward. Then Emma did the most incredible thing. She made a sort of bound in front of me, and almost knocked me back into the gutter. At the same moment I suddenly heard a growing noise and a car roared across the zebra ahead of me and up the road. Another inch forward, if Emma had not stopped me, and I would have been killed. The whole incident took only seconds, but when it happened I just stood there on the crossing, totally petrified. I heard the engine next to me stop and the sound of a cab door sliding open. Then the sound of an anxious voice. It was a corporation bus driver.

'Are you all right?'

'Yes,' I said.

'I've never seen anything like it. I couldn't get his number. He must have been doing fifty miles an hour.'

'Yes,' I said, still too shaken to react any more.

Then the driver added, 'I've never seen anything like your dog, either. It's lucky she did that. You've got a good dog there, lass.'

With that, he got back into his cab, started up and drove off. Emma, in turn, was anxious to be going, and as she trotted placidly along I kept thinking of the bus driver's words. Yes, I certainly did have a good dog. She had saved my life.

10

Emma's Operation

THE BLIND MOBILITY Research Centre at Nottingham University was always coming up with bright new ideas, and asking local blind people to help test them. One ingenious piece of work they did was to make a braille map of the new Victoria shopping centre. This, on the site of the old Victoria railway station, is an enormous place, two storeys high, with all the shops under cover, air-conditioned and set out amid fountains and flower gardens. It is splendid, but poses problems for the blind. There are no steps to count, no kerbs, and nothing by which people without sight can orientate themselves. So the Mobility Research Centre made a braille map, and put braille labels and notices round the shopping centre. The main area has large concrete pillars all the way down the middle. Numbers in braille were attached to each pillar. By feeling the number on a pillar and relating it to the equivalent number on the braille map, it became possible to know exactly which shops were nearby. The map was a brilliant construction – the entire centre on paper as a tactile image: lines drawn for the outlines of shops, pillars indicated in large round raised dots, stairs by little series of lines which gave an impression of stairs through the fingers.

It was decided to make a film of how the scheme worked, and I was asked if I would take part with Emma. Ian, the cameraman, briefed us on exactly what was expected in the filming, and what they wanted us to do. The idea was to make it look like a typical shopping day for a blind person, starting off in the bus station.

Geoffrey, who was directing the film, asked me if I had any idea how films were made, and I told him I knew about shooting and cutting in a vague sort of way, because I had read about it. 'Yes,' he said, 'that's it, we do all the shots, and then edit the film into the sequences we want. There's one thing, though: we might want a shot from different angles, so you may be asked to do something twice or three times. I hope that'll be OK, but it can get a bit tedious.' I promised I would try to make as few mistakes as possible.

Emma and I did as we were told for the beginning of this epic, and the cameras started turning. But we had not gone more than half a dozen paces when I was suddenly taken by the arm. 'Hello, I haven't seen you for some time. How's Emma getting on?' It was one of the bus inspectors who knew Emma and me. I heard Graham shout 'Cut!' After the inspector had chatted for a bit (I could not risk telling him we were making a film otherwise he would probably have wanted to be in it), we had another go. This time, Emma and I got as far as the door into the centre. And then I heard the sound of a great commotion. 'Why don't you look where you're going?' I heard someone say (and thought they meant me). Then: 'You can see she's blind can't you?' Ian, the cameraman, had run in close to get a better shot of me coming up to the door, and some of the shoppers thought he was going to collide with me, and took him by the arm. So, another length of film was ruined, and we had to start again. Emma, I could tell, was by now becoming rather fed up with doing the same run, but the take went reasonably well this time. Next I located the first pillar with the braille number, and stood reading my map, which was what they wanted to film. Almost immediately I heard a woman's voice, very close, 'Where do you want to go, my dear? I'll take you.' It was the kindest of gestures. But, in the background, I heard yet again 'Cut!' When she had gone we managed to do this shot properly.

The next location was more difficult. We had to go down to the north end of the centre and find a cafe where we were going to be filmed having a cup of tea. The trouble was, I could not find the pillars, and I had no means of asking Emma to find one for me. In any case, she had spent all her life trying to avoid such things and obviously was not going to learn a new trick now. So I had to listen for the pillars, then stop and feel, with my arm outstretched. It must have looked very strange. But at last I thought I had found a pillar, and put my arm out. This pillar, however, did not seem to be made of concrete. I realised I was grasping a handful of overcoat. The man concerned in this odd assault apologised to me for some reason. He must have thought I was mad.

On the next attempt we found the right pillar and had our cup of tea. The film was finished in the end, and I understand it turned out very well, with not a hint of the genuine drama that had gone into its making.

Round about this time, one aspect of life that was beginning to worry me a little was the fact that the flat had no garden for Emma to run in. It really came home to me one August day. I was sitting in the flat, knowing that outside it was glorious and sunny, and thought languidly how marvellous it would be to have a garden. There were parks not far away where I took Emma for her free run. But this was not the same as being able to open the door at any time and let her out. Nor was it the same as Emma having her own patch of lawn and her own boundaries. Sitting thinking about it, I had an idea. It was two months to Emma's birthday, 16 October, and a garden would be the best present I could give her. I went to the phone and rang the local housing department. The idea was to exchange my flat for a house.

They were not very helpful. The upshot of their response was that it was very unlikely that anyone would want to exchange a council house for the kind of flat we were in, but I was welcome to try and arrange it for myself, if I could. I tried, and had no success. Then I remembered that Emma had a friend on the council. She was a very kind woman called Brenda Borritt, who used to see us in the park quite often and took an interest in Emma. So the next time we met in the park I told her about the problem, and she said she would see what could be done. A week or two went by, and I was beginning to think that nothing would come of the idea, when there was a telephone call. Mrs Borritt had found someone who wanted to move out of their council bungalow into a flat. It was, she said, only a small bungalow, prefabricated and getting on in years – but it had a garden!

So Emma got her present: but only just in time. We moved house on the very day. Emma took to the house at once, and even more, to the garden. It was not very big. But there was enough space for her to go out whenever she wanted, with grass, and flower beds and rose trees.

It took the upheaval of moving house to bring home to me again that I could not see. This may sound odd.

But having Emma I never had the feeling when I went out that I was blind. Through Emma I could see: not in a visual sense, obviously, but I knew what was going on around me as she reacted to her surroundings. All her feelings and moods transmitted themselves through the harness. I could always tell if there was an obstacle ahead because of the way she slowed up and hesitated ever so slightly. I knew when we were passing another dog, because I could feel her looking, and her tail wagging.

But around the house it was different. Moving in a room, or from one room to another, a blind person is always mentally planning. And moving to a new house, you have to start all over again.

Don helped me move in, and we had a hectic time: he put up curtain rails and changed electric plugs, while I carried on the endless business of unpacking. Emma and I collapsed into bed at about two in the morning. In next to no time, it seemed, I heard someone knocking outside (it was, in fact, Don) and I quickly got out of bed. Then I realised I could not remember exactly where the door was. I felt along one wall, and then another, and opened a door. I was in a fitted wardrobe. After trying another wall, and coming back again to the fitted wardrobe I finally found the right door. Pausing only to collide with the settee that I had forgotten had been put in the middle of the living room, I got to the front door.

There was no one there. Then I remembered there was a back door as well, where Don was patiently waiting. It took me a long time to become accustomed to all the different doors, after being so used to my flat with its one entrance and fewer rooms.

That was not all. I remember going to the loo one day, and finding it was not there. I was in the wrong room, as I discovered after five minutes searching and feeling round for porcelain and a plastic seat. I even got lost in the garden, small as it was. I had left Emma in the kitchen and shut the back door as I went to hang out some washing. Then I lost my sense of direction completely, and could not remember where the back door was. I felt all round the hedges, and over the front gate, and back to the house before finally finding it. I wondered afterwards if Emma had been staring reproachfully at me through the window.

Emma, however, very soon got used to her garden. She could not wait to be let out, and used to gallop all over, snorting at the hedge bottoms on the trail of long-vanished cats.

Of course, not only the house, but the new area presented its problems. We had moved to the Beechdale district, and there were a lot of new routes to be learned, including a new one to work. Not long after we had moved into the new house, I had to go to Boots the Chemists to fetch a prescription. Emma knew Boots very well: it was in the main street of Nottingham, Parliament Street, on the left-hand side, and she took me there straight away after we had got off the bus. She took me up the steps to the door, and I put my hand out, but the door would not open. It was very odd, because Boots was normally open day and night. 'Are you sure,' I asked Emma, 'you've got the right place?' We came back down the steps, and, as I was turning over in my mind why they could possibly be closed, she took me along the pavement. I felt Emma turn to a crossing. When the traffic stopped we went over, and she took me up to a shop. I thought: 'Well, at least I can ask in here.' But when we got inside I heard a familiar voice. It was a Boots assistant, saying, 'Hello, Emma.' Then she said, 'I saw you across the road, and I was just coming over to fetch you. We've closed down over there. Then I saw Emma bringing you across, so I didn't bother. She certainly had a good look at the notice across the way saying we've closed!'

At the nearby Post Office, the woman soon got to know us, and became very fond of Emma. We used to go a lot, because I had my talking-books to post. Talking books are large cassettes that will not fit an ordinary tape recorder. They are played on a special machine. The service is a boon for the blind, and is run from Bolton, in Lancashire. The cassettes cover all kinds of books from classical works to light fiction, recorded by first-class readers, often from the BBC. The talking book library sends out its catalogue, available in ordinary print or braille, for a subscription of £3 a year, and about thirty books at a time can be chosen. These are then sent, two or three together, and this ensures that when a used cassette is sent back, there is another to listen to while the next batch is on its way. In this way I have 'read' widely from Jane Austen to James Bond.

There is one advantage in assimilating books in this way: I used to switch my book on, and carry on feeding Emma, washing over the kitchen floor and doing the ironing, and by the time I had finished I would be three chapters of the book further on.

The Post Office – another good service they perform for the blind – deals with the talking book traffic free of charge. The cassettes arrive in plastic cases, with a perspex square in the front. The address is on a card behind the perspex, and all that has to be done to return the cassette is to turn the card over and replace it. The library centre's address is on this reverse side.

People sometimes used to ask me how I knew if Emma was not well. Obviously I could not see whether she had a dry nose, had lost condition in her coat, or was lacking her normal bounce. But I did not need to see her. People did not appreciate the extraordinary bond between us. I could tell as soon as we got up in the morning, and she had her first vigorous shake, how she was, and even what kind of a mood she was in. She might be a little less enthusiastic than usual about going out to work, and, of course, even if I could not see her nose, I could always feel if it was warm. She might ask to go out into the garden more than usual. I could certainly tell if she was off colour.

In addition, because she was a guide dog (there is a little disc round her neck saying: 'I am a guide dog') she had a check-up every six months at the vet's. This is free of charge to the guide dog owner, and is a good plan for anticipating any trouble before it becomes serious. There was only one snag about this bi-annual ritual as far as Emma was concerned: she was not at all keen on the idea.

I had to be slightly devious for her own good. When preparing for a visit to the vet's I would never say anything to her, because Emma knew the street the surgery was in as a familiar route. Her pace always slackened on the approach to the vet's door, until she was hardly putting one paw in front of the other. Then, when she realised we were not actually making a visit, she would switch into top gear, and we would zoom past as if very late for an urgent appointment.

When the visit was a genuine one I am afraid I used to have to wait until poor Emma had just about come to a stop by the steps leading to the door, go up them, feel for the doorbell, hold on and use gentle force to get her over the mat.

She loathed it. But there came the day, in between the six-monthly check-ups, when I first felt a small lump under her chest. I kept a check on it, and it seemed to be growing, so I decided I would have to take her to the vet's. After we got over the inevitable dramatic performance on the doorstep, and the normal yelps and barks from other dogs as we waited, we found Mr Davidson on duty: a very kind man, a great lover of Labradors, and fond of Emma in particular.

He examined the lump and told me it had best be removed to be on the safe side. This meant I had to arrange to take Emma in early the following morning. Normally dogs that are operated on are left all day, but in our case I did not want this to happen. We agreed that if I could get a car to bring me to the surgery, she need stay only a couple of hours: I simply did not want her to be there long without me.

Of course I was terrified that the lump might be malignant. I told the girls at work, and they were immediately worried and sympathetic. They all agreed that once I had taken Emma in to the surgery, I ought to be picked up by a firm's car and taken home after the operation, and have the rest of the week off to look after her. It did not work out quite like that, but it was a kind thought.

The following morning I took Emma, protesting as ever, to the surgery, and after Mr Davidson had given her the anaesthetic, I stayed with her until she was asleep. One of the drivers from the garage, who were immensely kind and understanding about this whole business, took me in to work and I waited the two hours. My thoughts were in turmoil: terrible anxiety for Emma, mixed with anticipation of the problems that would be involved in getting about without her to lead me. The lump on her chest was just where the harness went, and she would certainly not be able to wear it for a little while at least. Those two hours were quite extraordinary. Not only was I worried because Emma was at the vet's under an anaesthetic, but I instinctively kept feeling her bed under the switchboard, listening for her, expecting to feel her touch my knee with her nose. It was like having left part of myself somewhere else. It was a very upsetting, empty feeling. I couldn't bear the thought of anything happening to Emma.

At last, twelve o'clock came and again my chauffeur from work took me down to the vet's, parked and waited for me to fetch Emma. I felt my way up the steps to the door with the help of the rail, rang the bell and was shown into the waiting room. Then Mr Davidson brought Emma in. She had not long recovered consciousness, and I could hear by her walk she was shaky on her feet. But her welcome! The way she wagged her tail was nearly making her fall over; I heard her slip and slide about as she saw me. Even in that state she made an immense fuss of me, bless her.

When I'd thanked Mr Davidson, I clipped her lead round her collar ring instead of putting her harness on, and we made our way out. I went very slowly, as much for my own sake as Emma's, but when the door was opened for us, Emma turned round and took hold of the lead about half-way up, and walked round in front of me. I was not very sure why, but then realised that we were at the top of the steps and she was telling me that because she was not wearing her harness, she could not help me in her normal way: so, instead, she was taking the lead in her mouth to guide me.

We got home, and Emma slept peacefully in front of the fire for most of the day while the anaesthetic wore off. But I was dreadfully worried, wondering what news would come about the lump. The waiting seemed endless. I had a nightmare that I was in the middle of Nottingham, alone, with no Emma and no Don, and there were people all around me, and noise and confusion. I could not move I was so terrified. Two days later, there was good news in the post: the results from the laboratory were negative. It had only been a fatty lump, and there was nothing malignant. My relief was boundless.

Emma had only a small wound, with about four stitches in it. But so that she would not scratch it, I decided to put part of a pair of tights over it. Emma must have looked very odd. I cut the legs off the tights, and made a hole in the gusset which was to go over her head, so that the body part went over her ribs and no dirt would get to the wound. It meant a new pair of tights for her every day, and when we came to fitting them, Emma was always delighted. I think she was quite proud of her new look.

During this period when Emma could not work, I felt quite helpless. I suppose I might have been able to get to the shops without Emma, but I really did not have the courage even to try to set foot outside the door without her. She had been with me for so long the idea was inconceivable.

Fortunately she was back in harness fairly soon, because the wound healed quickly. As we strode off down the street together it seemed incredible to be free again. And knowing what it was like without that freedom made the feeling even greater.

11

The Cats

SOON AFTER I moved into the new bungalow in Beechdale it struck me that, once again, I would be able to have a cat. There had not been a cat in our lives since Tiss, but now I would be able to fulfil an ambition: I should be able to have a Siamese cat. Ever since I had taken Emma to the vet one day, and we had sat next to someone with a litter of Siamese, I had wanted one. I had been given one of the kittens to hold, and I was struck by its delicate frame and elegance and length, quite apart from the uncannily human sound made by the litter.

So one evening I asked Don if he would look in the paper to see if there were any Siamese advertised. He kept looking until one night, after a spate of Jack Russells for sale, he came across what we wanted. 'Red point Siamese,' he said, 'what are they?'

'I've no idea, but they sound very attractive, don't they? What's the telephone number?'

I rang the breeder there and then and she described the cats to me as having golden-red ears, paws, tail and face, with sapphire blue eyes and an almost white body coat. They sounded gorgeous. So we made an appointment to go and inspect them. Emma came along, of course, for apart from having to take me there, she would also have to approve, or not, as the case might be. We chose a male kitten, four months old, and named him Ohpas, which is the Siamese for sunlight. We hadn't had him long before it was apparent he had fleas and other disorders and the vet's bills mounted alarmingly before eventually he was in good health. But this we did not know on the afternoon we brought him home.

When we arrived, I let him out of his little carrier, and he was so nervous of anything that moved that he went behind the armchair and would not budge. Nothing I could do would bring him out. Some hours later I was sitting down to dinner and just cutting into a juicy steak when I felt something climbing onto my knee: Ohpas, obviously. So to encourage him (mistakenly as I later realised) I cut a very small piece of meat and gave it to him. Almost immediately there was a rather more authoritative tap on my other knee. It was Emma. It had always been a rule that Emma never had titbits from the table. But what could I do? In fairness I had to cut her some, too. And in next to no time both my knees were under attack from alternate sides. Between them, Ohpas and Emma had most of the steak I had so been looking forward to. I did enjoy the grilled tomatoes, though. They were not interested in them.

The most marvellous thing about Ohpas was that he worshipped Emma. He used to sit on the settee and it became his job to wash her face and ears. Like Tiss, Ohpas seemed to know that Emma was something special among dogs, and this feeling was evident with every cat we had afterwards: it was a strange communication of knowledge between animals that the relationship between them and the human beings was clearly defined, and Emma's role and importance were unmistakable to the cats.

The absent-minded professor side to Ohpas's character was most evident when he fed. Siamese like to take their food to where *they* want to eat it, not necessarily eat from the bowl where it is provided. Ohpas was no exception, and he used to prefer to take his piece of meat into the living room, and sit in front of the fire eating it in comfort. His routine never varied. Don, once again, was able to describe to me exactly what happened. Ohpas would take the meat from the bowl, put it down on the hearthrug, and then fastidiously wash himself before settling to enjoy it. Unfortunately, Emma occasionally used to spy out what was happening, and since where food is concerned Emma can resist anything but temptation, the meat would be gone in a flash, and the air would be filled with a strange sort of pert, questioning mewing: 'I know I had a piece of meat, but where has it gone?' I would then be touched on the knee, and there would be more inter-rogative mewing: 'Do *you* know what's happened to my food?' The simple solution, of course, was to provide another piece of meat. But, just as often, Emma would be watching and waiting, nose on the carpet, like an alli-gator in the shallows, and the same thing would happen all over again.

When I bought a second Siamese, to keep Ohpas company, she too took instantly to Emma. She was a most intelligent and regal animal called Ming. Emma, in turn, recognising a likeable and kindred intelligence, almost immediately set to work moulding her into a partner in crime. Emma's besetting greed had only one major obstacle in the house. She was unable to reach up to and across the draining board. Ming was accordingly trained to come to the rescue. I have no idea how it was done. But plainly Emma taught her to get on to the draining board (with Siamese silence and stealth) and throw any scraps, or even more tasty prizes, down for Emma to eat. Don used to watch this extraordinary performance (when they were unaware they were being observed) and he told me that Ming was mainly concerned in getting the food to Emma, and reserved hardly a morsel for herself.

I used to feed them all separately, and Emma had the good grace never actually to steal from the bowls as the cats fed. But Ming always left a little, and when she walked away from her bowl, it was the signal for Emma to come in like a canine vandal falling on the fleshpots of Rome, and plundering not only what was left by Ming, but any remains that Ohpas had unwittingly overlooked.

Having one male, Ohpas, and one female, Ming, in the household produced an inevitable result: a litter of Siamese kittens. It came as no surprise. The evening Ming started producing her kittens, Don was not with me, and I had a horrible feeling that if anything did go wrong, I would have no idea what to do. But it all went off quite undramatically. First I heard a very small squeak, announcing that a kitten had arrived, and no sooner, it seemed, had I heard this little noise, than I felt Ming come along and put something on my foot. I put my hand down very cautiously, and I felt a moist, tiny ball of fur.

I was surprised, because I had always understood that cats were very possessive about their offspring. Therefore, in case Ming really was not quite sure what she was doing, I picked up the new arrival in a paper handkerchief so as not to get my scent on it, and returned it to Ming. But shortly afterwards there was another minute noise, and Ming brought her second kitten out to me ... then a third ... and the entire routine was performed five times.

So, there I was with a litter of five! After three weeks I had the business of weaning them, and this was slightly more difficult for me. The principle is to take some patent milk, the kind used for babies, make it up, put a little finger in and let the kittens take it from the finger. My trouble was that it was hard to find their mouths, and sometimes they had milk applied to the ear! But we managed.

It wasn't long before I decided I should like to show the Siamese, which may sound the ultimate in lunacy. Still, I decided I would try it. Friends came to the rescue, and in spite of not being able to see, I learned how to groom the cats and how to know by touch whether they were perfectly clean. Ohpas, being white, tended to collect dirty marks, but here Don would help and point out offending spots which I would then clean. His ears I would do with cotton wool, and, once again, Don would inspect them. The details of my travels with the cats would require a book in themselves, but suffice it to say that the hall is now full of rosettes and commendations from shows all over the country.

In the event, showing Ohpas became less of a problem than that of the rising generation: Ming's five kittens. As they began to grow up, I really wondered what I had unloosed. Siamese are not only possessed of berserk inclinations, they are delinquent to an extreme degree. They zoomed up and down curtains and round and round the living room at sixty miles an hour, over tables, chairs and mantelpiece but never the floor; they were rather like a miniature but lethal chapter of Hell's Angels roaring round.

I constantly had to make excuses for them. Don came to see me one evening and said in surprise, 'I didn't know you were going to start stripping the wallpaper.' Because I really thought he might not approve, I had to say that, in fact, I had suddenly thought the bathroom needed redecorating; needless to say, it had been Ming's dreadful brood that had been responsible.

The trouble with all these games, which I could not see, but which I knew were going on, was that I had no idea where each of them had got to at any given moment, and it worried me sometimes. Every so often I had to have, so to speak, a roll call. I had learned to recognise by touch every one of the kittens, which was pleasing, because apparently they were difficult to tell apart visually. But I was able to distinguish between them either by their slightly differing weights, or by the shape of their heads, or by the length of their bodies and their tails.

At about this time a new anxiety about Emma was beginning to emerge. Once a year she had to be passed fit to do her work by the Guide Dog Association. She was due for a check in January 1975, and because she was over ten years old I was a little concerned. I began to fear that she might be retired simply on the grounds of her age. Such a lot of my friends who had guide dogs of about that age were being advised to retire them and go for new dogs. I could not bear the thought. I would often talk about it to Don, and he would say, 'Oh, there's no need to worry. Even if she had to retire I can take her with me to the surgery every day. She'll be all right. She'll be quite happy.' Well, possibly she might, I thought, but it was a terrible, desolating prospect to have to face.

I knew that I would not really be losing Emma, but the idea of any other dog doing her job, of being in harness with me, seemed so disloyal. It was unthinkable. I remembered all those years ago, my first evening at the training centre and how Dotty had wept, and, faced with the same situation myself, I really understood how heartbroken she had felt at having to go for a replacement for her first dog.

I could not bear to have the partnership broken. Emma was such a part of me. But the letter from the Guide Dog Association said that the trainer would arrive on Thursday at two o'clock, and I was dreading what he might say, even though rationally I knew that Emma worked as well as any younger dog, was sprightly, on her toes and as full of energy as she had ever been.

The trainer not only checks that the dog is fit, but also makes sure that the guide dog owner is helping to make it a team effort, and that no slipshod habits have crept in since his previous visit. So I wondered, too, how I would make out, though the thought was unimportant beside my concern for Emma.

He arrived on the dot of two, and Emma was on her best behaviour as I put her harness on and braced up to the task, and I hoped so much that he would not see anything that I had not been able to detect in her work. 'I'll go through town,' I said, 'if it's all right with you; it's our usual route to the bus station.'

The trainer was a pleasant man called Mr Soames, and he said that was fine. We had not picked the best of days. There was a great wind that beat against us when we set off and shortly there was a flurry of snow in our faces. But we carried on towards the bus stop, and Emma seemed the least troubled of any of us. She trotted along the pavement in her normal fashion. Then at one busy crossing I could hear two dogs growling and barking at each other, and I hoped nothing would happen. Emma ignored them completely and crossed right by them.

As we went along, I realised again how she loved working in town. She was weaving in and out of the people on a busy pavement, across the controlled cross-ings without a moment's hesitation as the bleeping sound went, and she seemed to have put on an even faster pace than usual. By the time we were at the bus stop and the end of the test, I was exhausted.

I waited for the decision. I had half made up my mind that if it went against us I was going to say I refused to have Emma retired. Then Mr Soames said, 'I saw Emma about four or five years ago.'

'Oh, did you?' I said, wondering where this was leading.

'Yes. You haven't been putting brown boot polish on her nose have you?'

'Boot polish, no, of course not.' (What was he driving at, what was he going to say?)

'Well, it's very strange. She hasn't gone a bit grey you know.'

'I know, everyone tells me she's not at all grey, and still looks very young.'

'She does,' said Mr Soames, 'she does look very young.'

I just had time to begin thinking: 'He's leading up to tell me that she looks young, but he knows that she's getting on in years' … when he said, 'No, she hasn't changed a bit. She really doesn't look a day older than when I last saw her.'

'No,' I said.

But Mr Soames did not say any more, and I suddenly grasped his meaning.

'You mean,' I said, 'you're not going to tell me to retire her?'

'Retire her?' he said, sounding quite surprised. 'Retire Emma? No, no, of course not. Goodness me.' Then he laughed. 'I should think the way she's shown us all up today she'll still be working when she's eighteen!'

It was like the sun suddenly coming out and shining on my face: marvellous. I said goodbye to Mr Soames, and Emma and I set off home. On the way back I stopped to buy her a new rubber bone. And that evening Don and I went out to celebrate.

Not long after this we had an even greater cause for happiness. At long last all the uncertainty, the lonely nights and five years of waiting were over. Don was free to marry me.

Yet I did not want to rush out to tell the world and have a big elaborate wedding. I felt that our love was a very private thing, and I wanted to share it with only very close family and a friend or two. When I called to invite them, they were absolutely thrilled at the news.

'What shall I wear?' I asked Don.

'Well, love, it's up to you, it really is.'

'It's got to be something green,' I said, because I associated green with spring, and with all things that were fresh and lovely.

The next day I went shopping with my mother. She searched through countless dresses before selecting one that she liked the look of, and I liked the feel of. But there was Emma to consider, too. I thought that perhaps she ought to have a bow. But then Don and I decided it would not be dignified for our maid of honour.

The day finally came. It was cold as Emma and I sat in the taxi on the way to the registry office, but I could feel the sun warm on my face, like the feeling I had inside. Emma had been given special permission to attend, particularly because I had pointed out that I refused to be married without her.

I found I was trembling as I pushed open the heavy door. I could not believe it was happening, that Don would be mine forever. Inside, I heard his voice call out, 'Hello, darling.' He took my hand. 'You look beautiful,' he said.

As Don held my hand, I felt he was trembling too, and I could hardly say the simple words 'I will' in front of the registrar. Emma must have sensed the extreme tension, for halfway through the service her cold, wet nose nuzzled my left hand, as if in moral support.

Then it was all over, and Don and I walked out hand in hand. I felt the confetti and my mother and father embrace me, but I don't think I was really aware of what was happening around me, or even what had in fact happened, until I heard Graham come up. He said, 'Well, Sheila, it's Mrs Hocken at last.' Then I knew it was really true. I did not have to pinch myself to see if I was in fact dreaming.

Yes, I said to myself, thinking flirtingly of my old assumption that I would never marry. *Mr and Mrs Hocken.* It was what mattered most in the world. And at the little bungalow that was now our home, the corks popped far into the night in celebration of that joyous fact.

12

Fresh Hope

ONE BLEAK JANUARY day in 1975, Emma and I had just come in after doing some shopping on the way back from work, and as I put the key in the latch of the front door I heard the telephone ringing. For some reason the key did not work properly, and I remember tugging and turning it impatiently and hoping the phone would not stop. When I finally got inside and lifted the receiver, I heard my brother Graham's voice.

Graham, as I've mentioned, has a similar eye complaint to mine, but despite having lost the use of one eye entirely because of a bad piece of surgery when he was very young, he always had, unlike me, some residual vision. In addition, he was constantly seeking means to improve the sight he had. He was ringing now to tell me about his latest efforts. He had gone to a new optician in order to try and get some contact lenses, and the optician had advised him to go and see a specialist called Mr Shearing, with the advice: 'This man is really good. There are a lot of new techniques that he knows all about. Go and see him.'

So, despite the reluctance of our family in general, and Graham in particular, to have anything to do with specialists or eye surgery because of bitter experience in the past, Graham had gone to see Mr Shearing who was an ophthalmic surgeon.

I was excited on his behalf; and almost before Graham could say 'Hello' I was asking, 'How did you get on? What happened?'

'Well,' he said, 'good news and bad news. He said it would be fairly simple to operate and remove the lens that my cataract is on, but in my case, he wouldn't really like to take the risk because there's only something like an eighty-five per cent success rate. Because I've got some vision he said it would be a terrible thing if the op wasn't successful. He wants me to wait a bit longer to see if anything new develops; anyway, the older I am the easier the operation is, because as you know, the lens hardens off with age, and the easier it is to break and bring away without any danger of messing up the rest of the workings of the eye.'

I felt a bit deflated, but then he went on, 'But I did think that you could go and see him. He's a very nice sort of chap, practical but extremely sympathetic. You never know what he might be able to do for you.'

And it struck me that Graham was right. What would

be the harm in just going and putting my case to this specialist? I rang up the following day and made an appointment, and I was quite surprised, when I put the phone down, to find that I felt quite shaky.

I suppose the reason was that I had always, on a conscious level, accepted the fact of going blind. But underneath, like all blind people, I had *never* accepted it. There is always a small voice somewhere at the back of the mind insisting: 'I've got to see. I can't go on living like this.' But that voice always has to be strangled, suppressed, put out of mind, because if you heed its message you will never be anything more than a ragbag of regret, and unable to take your part in the world, a part limited by the fact that you can't see.

I think that to make the most of that part is the only possible way to survive as a blind person. I'm always distressed when I meet people who have lost their sight and never bothered to learn braille. I say 'never bothered', but it is the wrong phrase. If I said they were 'unable' that would also be wrong. What is behind their attitude is a dogged, misguided lack of acceptance of the facts as they are. They prefer to dream instead. They are so convinced that they are going to have their sight restored somehow. Their conversation is always of the last specialist they went to, or the operation they are going to have, or, worse, 'They say that the next opera-tion might …' and 'They hope that in a few years …' It is all so understandable, but so sad, because such active hopes simply prevent the day-to-day business of getting on with life on the terms that have been dictated. I always tried to work along the lines of acceptance. It was only when I thought of the possibility of having sight again, that the frustration and sheer hatred of being blind arose. And here I was, trembling, because those very hopes were rising in me.

I had to wait three weeks before going to see Mr Shearing. The hopes got bigger, the hatred of blindness more intense. My imagination ran riot. When I made the appointment I said to Don, 'Well, that's it. Isn't it fabulous? I'm going to start saving. I'll be able to buy a car – I'll be able to go anywhere I want.' The idea of having to pass a test never even entered my head. I went on, 'I'll be able to join the public library, I can't wait to go round all those shelves. I'll be able to read anything I choose.'

'Yes,' said Don, 'marvellous.' But at the same time, his voice did not sound as enthusiastic as it might have done.

'What's the matter?' I said.

Then he tried to tell me as tactfully and gently as he could, in effect, not to build my hopes up too much. He wanted to be encouraging but he did not want me to be let down if things didn't work out. I knew what he was saying. I heard his words, which were meant to protect me. Yet I still could not stop dreaming. I let my excitement get the better of me. Yes, it might not work. But *what if it did*? It was a prospect I could not resist. It must have been a difficult time for Don, not wanting to pour cold water on my hopes, yet so afraid for me if what I most wanted in the world did not come about.

And during the three interminable weeks that I had to wait for the appointment with Mr Shearing, my imagination ranged over the countless possibilities of what sight would mean to me. At last the Friday came for my appointment. Graham said he would come with me because we had to go a long way, and even with Emma he thought it might be difficult for me to find my way round the unfamiliar streets. In truth, I think he wanted to come with me anyway. He wanted to be the first to know what went on: he had a vested interest in the outcome of the interview.

We agreed to meet at the bus station. I had told Emma we were going to meet Graham (she knew the names of all my friends and close relatives) and when we arrived, I knew she had spotted him. Her tail began to wag, tickling the palm of my hand, and she quickened her pace, took me on, stopped and sat down.

I heard Graham's voice as we approached. 'Hello, you're early. The bus isn't in yet.'

'Mm, I know. I wasn't going to miss it, so I left plenty of time.'

Then I heard the bus coming in. Emma led me on and found a seat for me, then, as always, lay quietly under the seat, while Graham sat down next to me. Graham is not a great one for small talk and chat, so we sat there not saying anything much as the bus moved off. It was an hour's journey from Nottingham, and as we left the echoes of the bus station behind and started off through the traffic I felt excited, and all sorts of thoughts about the possibility of seeing began to stalk through my mind. I suddenly thought about Emma, and for the first time, my worries about having to have another dog because of Emma's age were quietened.

It was the first time that I realised that if I could see, she would not have to guide me; I would be able to take her for a walk like other dogs, the partnership of nine years with all it meant would not have to be wrenched apart. It was a wonderful possibility.

Graham led the way to the consulting rooms, then said he would leave me there because he had some shopping to do. We rang the bell, and he said, 'I'll be back in about half an hour. All the best.'

The door opened, and I smelt that strangely clean and antiseptic smell mixed with floor polish that belongs to doctors' houses. A receptionist led me into the waiting room, and I sat there alone, Emma beside me. I was not there very long before I heard the door open, and a quiet voice said, 'Mrs Hocken?' I stood up. 'Would you come this way, please?' Emma guided me through the waiting room, across a very narrow hall, and into what sounded to me like a very big room with fitted carpets. I felt a fire in front of me; Emma had headed for it straight away.

'Well, lassie,' I heard a voice say, 'what can I do for you?'

'I want to know if you can possibly help me.'

There was a silence during which I could hear the clock ticking somewhere away to my left, and the gas fire hissing. I realised afterwards that Mr Shearing must have had something of a surprise to see someone led into his consulting room by a guide dog: on the face of it, possibly a no-hope case.

Then, at last, 'Mm. Well. Would you care to sit down?'

I told Emma to find a chair. I felt it, took her harness off and sat down.

'What's your name, then, lassie?'

I thought, what a terrible memory, he can't even remember my name. 'Sheila Hocken,' I said.

'No, no. This lovely creature sitting beside you.'

'Oh,' I said, 'Emma.'

'Emma. Yes. That suits you.' And I heard him patting her. He went on, 'I used to have two boxers, you know.'

'Boxers? I love boxers.' I asked him about them, and he told me all the details. They had died of old age.

'Haven't you a dog now?'

'Mm. I've got a bloodhound. Very wilful blood-hounds are, you know, very wilful.'

I was enjoying talking about dogs, but was beginning to wonder if we were skirting round the main topic because it was difficult, and he could not bring himself to ask the questions. I was becoming nervous, but at last he asked me to tell him all about my eyes.

I explained about the hereditary factor, and how his seeing my brother and holding out a wonderful opportunity for him had led me to come along. He was very quiet as I went on.

When I had finished he led me over to another chair and put drops in my eyes to dilate the pupils so that he could make a better examination. 'I'll leave you here for a little while so that can work. I'll be back in about ten minutes.' I heard him go out of the room and close the door behind him. Once again all I could hear was the clock, and the hiss of the gas fire, with, this time, Emma's sleeping deep breaths added, keeping up an odd counterpoint with the tick of the clock. I could hear nothing from outside, and in the air I could smell just the faintest aroma of cigar smoke.

He came back in what seemed to me less than ten minutes. I felt him examining my eyes. He hummed and ha'd a bit, and then said decisively, 'Right, come and sit in a more comfortable chair.' He led me back to where

I had been sitting before, and I heard him making a fuss of Emma again, and from her little snorts and growls I knew she was enjoying it. I was longing to ask him what he had seen, what he thought. But he just went on talking to Emma, telling her how beautiful she was. I almost became impatient, but sat and waited.

'Well, lassie,' he said finally. 'What do you expect I'm going to say?'

What did I expect? I didn't know. I couldn't think. It was too overwhelming even to frame into words the possibility I so much wanted to hear. I said, 'I don't know. I was hoping, after my brother had been to see you ...'

'Well,' said Mr Shearing, 'you know you've got cataracts. But you're aware of this retina problem, aren't you?'

I did know about the retina problem, but such is human nature, I had pushed this uncomfortable and depressing thought to the depths of my mind in the past few weeks. Such had been the power of the very idea of sight, I had virtually forgotten about it. But I remembered now.

'Yes,' I said rather lamely, 'I do remember that. But what does it entail? Could you explain it?'

'I'll have to try. Now, you have cataracts, and obviously we're talking about congenital cataracts, where the retina, depending on the thickness of the cataracts, has not had a proper chance to develop. The thicker the cataracts, the less chance of the light reaching the retina, and the less chance the retina has of developing properly.

'If the cataracts are very thick, the light can't get to the back of your eye, and as this has happened in your case, your retinas won't have developed.'

'Yes,' I said, my heart already sinking, 'I understand. But isn't there anything you can do?'

He sat there for what seemed an age. I felt my mind becoming cold and empty, and strangely numb. I was incapable of rational thought, or any reaction beyond suddenly wanting to get up and go, and not hear what he had to say.

But then, to my utter surprise, he said, 'Yes. I think there is. At least I could have a try. I could try removing the lens, or part of the lens, and see what success we have.'

Well, this was it, I thought. But I went in on the wave of sharp excitement too quickly. I said immediately, 'What sort of sight would I have? How much would I be able to see?'

And his reply brought me straight back to earth, and sitting in the chair bounded by darkness. 'It's a terribly difficult question, lassie. I just don't know.'

'Well,' I said, because I had to know as much as it was possible to know, despite the consequences, 'if you did an operation and it was a success, would I still need Emma to guide me? Would I be able to read for instance?'

'Oh,' he said, 'I think you'd still need Emma, and as for reading, well, lassie, I don't work miracles.'

I was desolate. All those thoughts of what I would – not even might – be able to do. I had expected a miracle, and should have known better.

He was a very gentle and kind man, Mr Shearing, and he must have seen the disappointment in my face. He said in a voice full of compassion, 'Now, lassie, I couldn't promise you anything. You wouldn't want a promise from me that you yourself knew might not be fulfilled. We might give you some sight, we might not. Well, it would be worth a try, wouldn't it? Anything would be better than what you have at the moment, don't you agree?'

Of course, he was right. 'Yes,' I said, 'anything at all would be better than nothing. I've got nothing to lose.'

When I asked him why Graham's case held out the possibility of perfect sight, he explained that my brother's cataract was very slight compared with mine, and the retinas were not retarded. He went on to say that my retinas, because of underdevelopment, would not pick up detail. They simply lacked the facility.

But by then, I knew I had to try for what might be possible. I said, 'Well, I must come in for an operation.'

'There's no need to rush into it, lassie. Go home, think about it and let me know on Monday.'

I felt utterly dejected. When Mr Shearing had gone, Graham said, 'Well?'

'Well – nothing.'

'Nothing? What do you mean? He must have said something.'

We walked back to the bus station and I told Graham more or less everything that had passed between me and Mr Shearing.

Graham gave a great sigh. 'What a terrible shame. I thought maybe you would stand to gain almost perfect sight.'

'Well,' I said, 'obviously not.'

'What are you going to do?'

'I'm going to have the operation.' I got on the bus, and Emma went to sleep under the seat as we rumbled back to Nottingham, and neither Graham nor I spoke.

When Don came home he tried to comfort me, but I sat there feeling sentenced for life. Until that afternoon there had always existed some hope that one day things might be better. But those last few hours had seemed to crush that possibility down so that though it did still exist, it seemed more of a formality to prove that it was not there at all, and never had been.

I had to have the operation, but I also had to face the strong possibility I would be blind for the rest of my life.

Then Don came to the rescue. He reminded me that when I was much younger I had been to eye specialists when I could see a little, and they had forecast that I would be totally blind. But though they had been nearly right – and right for all practical purposes – what they had meant was an utter black void, whereas I could still distinguish darkness from light. It was of no use to me. But I could. And the thought began to cheer me. What if Mr Shearing was wrong, too? In any case, I thought, no specialist is really going to promise a miracle. Miracles happened, but to promise them would mean they would never happen. So when I went to bed I was a little more cheerful, because of Don's love and encouragement. On Monday I rang Mr Shearing and said I would have the operation, and when I put the phone down, my hopes were still alive.

13

Hospital

I WAS TOLD that I might have to wait up to a year before the operation could be performed. In the event, the letter telling me it was all arranged arrived in September, so the delay was cut to a little under nine months. But they were nine months I never wish to live through again.

When the letter did arrive, it gave me only four days' notice, and this was a relief. I had to organise everything so quickly for my stay in hospital that there were few moments left over for further brooding or yearning. I was to go in on Wednesday, 3 September. The day before was a little like the last day of an old year, when one keeps thinking: 'This is the last time I shall do this in nineteen-seventy-whatever.' At the office everyone wished me luck, and one of the girls came up to me and said, 'Well, wait till you come back, you'll be able to see us all. I wonder what you'll think?'

'I don't know,' I said, 'won't it be marvellous?' She

was more confident than I was. With me, it was an enormous hope, not a certainty. But I could not pretend that I had not thought countless times about the visual identities of the people I knew so well by their voices. I had an impression of all their personalities, and what the office was like, and I had my own images of what everything and everybody looked like, but it was odd to think that I might be walking out of there for the last time as a blind person.

When I got home, I heard Emma lap at her bowl of water, then patter off into the living room, and thought: 'That might have been the very last time you had to take me anywhere, Emma.' Then I followed her, sat down and started thinking of the final practical details involved in going into hospital.

Don, of course, would be looking after Emma. He was going to take her to the surgery with him, and she would accompany him in the car on his rounds and wherever he went. Because of the short notice the hospital had given, there had been no chance to arrange time off for him to take me in, and obviously he could not cancel his patients. Instead, Deirdre, a friend of mine who was a nurse, was going to take me.

The following morning we were up early, and, thank goodness, the practicalities prevented most thoughts and feelings beyond a slightly nervous sensation in the pit of my stomach. Before Don went, I said, 'Now you won't forget to give Emma her biscuits, will you? Oh, and don't forget her bowl of milk in the morning ...'

Don replied patiently, 'Now you know I'll look after Emma. Don't worry. She's almost as much a part of me as she is of you.'

And I knew that was true. Then he kissed me, and said, 'Well, the best of luck.' I said something flippant, like 'I'll need it.' But the words only masked the feelings that we knew were overwhelming us both. Just as he was taking Emma out of the door, I said, 'I don't know how I'm going to face it without the pair of you to back me up.'

'Now don't *worry*,' said Don. 'Everything will be all right. And I'll be there every night.'

With that, he and Emma were gone. I heard the car start up, move away, and I felt so alone. I had never been parted from Emma in nine whole years, except when she had her operation, and that was only for two hours. Without Don and his constant reassuring presence any idea that the operation *might* be a success ebbed away.

Fortunately, Deirdre was not long in arriving, and she was full of kindness and remarks that restored my confidence. My suitcase was already packed. We chatted happily as we drove along. At the hospital she checked me in and took me to the ward, and left me with the same words as Don had used. 'Well, the best of luck.'

'Thanks Deirdre,' I said.

I was met at the ward by a young student nurse, a very pleasant girl called Jasmine. 'Oh yes. Mrs Hocken,' she said, 'would you like to come this way?' The sound of her footsteps then began to recede, and I thought: 'Help, what do I do?' She obviously didn't know I could not see, and so I stood there, feeling rather foolish, and wondering who was looking at me. Then I heard her coming back, and I explained, and I think she was more embarrassed than I was. I put out my hand to take her arm to go down the ward to my bed.

As we walked along, in addition to all my other feelings, I knew I did not like hospitals. I had a fear of them. I had not been in one since I was a child, and I still imagined them as sombre places with power over life and death. Fortunately, in the next few days, these gloomy ideas were rapidly dispelled. When we reached my bed, Jasmine asked if I would get undressed.

'Can you manage?' she asked.

'Yes, thanks,' I said, and added, 'do I have to get into bed?'

'Oh, no,' said Jasmine, 'just put your dressing gown on. Patients only go to bed at night here, because there's no one really ill. You can stay in the ward, if you like, or go into the day room.'

'Marvellous,' I said.

Then she began, 'What about magazines ...' and stopped herself with, '... oh, I am sorry, you can't read, I really am sorry.'

'That's all right,' I said, 'but I can read. I've brought some braille magazines with me.'

Jasmine, as it turned out, had never seen braille before, and was fascinated. She watched my fingers as I read from one of the magazines, and explained a bit about how braille works, with its contractions and abbreviations.

'Well,' she said, 'I don't think I could do that,' and took me down the ward to the day room. On the way, she showed me round the ward so that I could feel my way about, and get to know how many steps there were from my bed to the bathroom, how many beds were on each side of the ward, and so on.

In the day room there was a completely different atmosphere from that which I had expected. It was very friendly, homely almost, and everyone was surprised that I could not see, and had virtually never been able to. Most of the patients were older people who had come in to have cataracts removed, and, as a result, some of them were very troubled by their failing eyesight, and could not get about too easily. Having been so used to seeing perfectly in the past, they suffered a great deal, and I soon realised that I was, in effect, the least inconvenienced of them all.

I had two days to wait before my operation: the Wednesday of my arrival, and the Thursday. Mr Shearing came to see me on the second day, and stayed for a little while in the course of his normal rounds. I knew he was in the ward because of the faint aroma of cigar smoke which penetrated from beyond the doors: he must always have gone into Sister's office to have a cigar. He explained a little more to me about the operation, what had been done in the past, and what the newer techniques of eye surgery entailed. With a young patient the cataract is relatively soft and sticky (whereas with an older person it will have hardened off) and attempts had been made to make holes through the lens or pull part away, often resulting in detachment of the retina. Even when this had not happened, holes had been made in the lens which healed up as a scab and so the patient ended in a worse state than when he had gone into hospital.

Mr Shearing explained that he intended to take the middle part of my lens away. The lens, he said, was like an onion, with layer after layer of tissue, so taking the middle part away and leaving the outside would protect the retina, and let the light through the middle. He had no idea, of course, what my retina would be like, beyond the fact that it would not be developed, and it was believed that with this kind of retina detailed vision was an impossibility.

It was marvellous to talk to him, and though it still did not make me any the less scared, I had a kind of confidence in him. Don came in to see me on both evenings, and on the Thursday night he sat there and I remember saying, 'Well, this time tomorrow, it will all be over.'

'Yes,' said Don, not concealing his anxiety very well, 'I'll be thinking of you all tomorrow.'

Beyond that, not much passed between us apart from talking about what Emma had been doing, and how good she had been going round with Don in the car. For most of the time we just sat there and sort of hoped together.

I went to sleep very easily that night, and then, on Friday morning, woke up with a quite extraordinary feeling of being on top of the world. All the worries seemed to have disappeared. I knew this was the day, yet instead of being scared, I simply thought: 'Marvellous, I'm glad it's here, and I'm not worried. Marvellous.'

This was before the pre-med, even. At about nine o'clock I was taken down to the operating theatre, and although it seemed a long way, I still could not get over this feeling. It was not happiness as such, but a great feeling that something really momentous was about to happen, and that I need not be afraid. In the anteroom the anaesthetist gave me a final injection, and I remember simply trailing off thinking: 'This is the moment ... the moment of ...' and the words never materialised.

I came round in the ward. It would be about half-past four in the afternoon. My first thought was: 'It's over, thank goodness, it's over.' But I knew I would be bandaged over the eyes, so I was not expecting to be able to know immediately whether the operation had worked, and I remember thinking: 'I shall know soon enough.' But, most of all, I was feeling thirsty. I felt as if I could have drained a reservoir. Yet was not able to muster the effort to ask for a drink. I lay there, vaguely hearing other people coming and going and the now familiar sound of screens being wheeled and other hospital noises. After about an hour, I at last pulled myself round enough to say, 'Could I have a drink, please?'

Don was coming in to see me that evening, and I remember making a great effort not to be doped, and somehow to appear reasonably sensible and alert for him. I would know when he had arrived, by his footsteps approaching the bed. But all I heard were the nurses' footsteps, all different: Annette, Ann, Jasmine, Alison, Linda and Sister herself. Sister was a tremendous character who had not been there on the day I arrived. Sisters make or break a hospital ward, and this one certainly made it. Far from being a fire-breathing martinet, she spread an infectious goodwill. Her entrance into the ward was like uncorking champagne. She exploded into the ward, and bubbled all over. She kept everyone laughing and joking, and made it really a marvellous place to be in.

When I finally recognised Don's footsteps coming down the ward it was suddenly reassuring. His presence quieted the thoughts perpetually at the back of my mind: 'Has it worked? Hasn't it worked?'

Don sat by me and asked, 'When will they take the bandages off? When will you know?'

I said, 'Monday', and we both knew what an interminable time the weekend was going to seem.

It passed, as all time passes, however. My mother and father came in to see me on the Saturday, and my brother Graham, and all of us were facing possibilities we couldn't translate into adequate phrases.

'I bet you can't wait until Monday.'

'No, I can't.'

So much was unspoken behind this exchange. A family history of blindness – of pain and hope.

Don, when he came in again, could not hide his feelings and was very protective, saying, 'Well, you know, if it hasn't worked and you can't see, it won't matter as far as we're concerned, will it? It's never made any difference in the past, and there are still so many things to do together.'

It was such a kind and loving reassurance, trying to armour me against the worst possibility, and it took a lot for him to say it because it really meant so much to him as well as to me.

Time went on slowly in the ward, spaced out by the set hours for meals, temperature-taking, pills and sleep. On Sunday evening, Don was by my bedside again. We were sitting talking (I had been able to get up the morning after the operation), and he said, 'Now, you'll ring me, won't you?'

'Of course.'

'As soon as you know.'

'Of course I will.' I knew that he wanted so much to be there at the time the bandages were taken off, and to know as soon as I did, but it was impossible because of his practice.

When it was time for him to go, he said, 'Oh, I hope it's worked, I hoped it's worked …' Then, after a pause, he added, '… they're such insufficient words, aren't they?'

'No, they're not,' I said, 'I know just what you mean. The next time you come in, we really shall know.'

And from then, from the time that he went on the Sunday night, there began seemingly endless hours of waiting, an interminable countdown to the conclusion I could not escape.

The hours from eight o'clock Sunday evening to ten o'clock Monday morning would normally go in a flash, a brief interval from supper to going to work. But now time seemed stretched on the rack, and I with it. The minutes and seconds went on, and on, and on. I kept feeling my watch. I could hear it clicking away, but never fast enough.

In the bed on one side of me was May, and on the other Muriel. Both had been watchful and kind as I had been coming round, and I heard Muriel, quite late, call over to me, 'I can hear you feeling your watch. Don't worry. Morning will be here soon enough, you know. Try and get some sleep, Sheila.'

But sleep was out of the question. I felt my watch again. It was seven minutes past twelve. Past midnight. It was Monday! ... now my watch told me it was ten past one, then eight minutes to two, and then I think I did at last sleep a little, because next it was six o'clock, and the nurses were coming round and taking temperatures, and bringing the early tea.

I sat up. Another four hours, I thought, four whole hours. I lit a cigarette, which was not strictly permitted, but I was so strung up I hardly cared. Perhaps because everyone realised what I was going through no one asked me to stop smoking, which gave some relief at least.

At eight o'clock – several cigarettes later – breakfast came. I did not want it, but I thought: 'I must eat it. It will pass the time. It will take another fifteen minutes away.' All too soon I was down to the toast and marmalade, and it was still only ten past eight. What, I thought, am I going to do for nearly another two hours?

Muriel came over and asked, 'Are you all right?'

I said, 'Yes, I'm fine, but I think I shall go mad before ten o'clock. I just can't wait, it's terrible.'

'Why don't you go and have a bath? That'll fill in some of the time.'

'That's a good idea,' I said, and began searching in my locker for my various things. If I have a bath, I thought, it might take half an hour away if I take my time. But, though I thought I was being leisurely, I found that I took only about ten minutes. I must have been hurrying without noticing it.

When I got back in the ward I began pacing up and down, and again Muriel came over, and said, 'Do you want to go to the day room? We can go in there and listen to the radio.'

'No,' I said, 'I don't think I want to go down there, thanks all the same.'

The reason was that the dressing room where my bandages would be removed was just outside the door of the ward, but the day room was right at the opposite end, and at ten o'clock I wanted to be as near as I could to hear my name called.

So, in such a kind way, Muriel and May offered to bring a table up to my bed so that we could all sit there, and pass the time that way. Muriel, particularly, was marvellous in trying to keep my mind off the approaching, overwhelming question mark.

I said to her as we sat there, 'What's it like outside the ward? You know, what does it look like?' It was hard for me to form an idea of what the outside was like, and she described the scene to me, telling me about the many trees (which I could hear rustling outside the window). She also spoke of the roses growing outside, and this, all at once, like the touching of some secret spring, sent me away into another daydream. What was the ward like? I knew how many beds there were, and I knew that there were flowers by the beds and on the tables. Muriel in fact had said, 'Your flowers are nice', only that morning. I had some dahlias, but I had never been keen on dahlias. They felt spiky to me, and had no scent. I could not imagine them at all, unlike roses, or carnations, or hyacinths, each of which had its own special character through its perfume. I had no image of my dahlias, and I was, though it might seem ungrateful, hardly interested in them at all.

Every five minutes I kept feeling my watch, and, in between, I smoked endlessly. Muriel lectured me in a friendly sort of way about the amount I was smoking. I said, 'I know I shouldn't, but I must do something.' It was twenty to ten by then, and I had to get up and walk up and down again. My stomach kept turning over, and I was in a terrible state; always at the back of my mind there was that warning from Mr Shearing, 'I don't perform miracles, lassie.'

Then I heard Annette coming down the ward, and I called to her, 'Have you started the dressings yet?'

'Not yet,' she said, 'but we shan't be long ... and don't worry, we'll make sure you're first.' I felt my watch again. The dots must have been nearly worn away. There were only ten minutes to go.

14

The Bandages Come Off

WHEN AT LAST Sister came into the ward and called, 'Sheila', the strange thing was that nothing happened. I just sat there. Everyone has heard of people being paralysed with fear, or apprehension, or whatever, and I suppose this is literally what happened. I was sitting just inside the ward, not more than a few yards from the dressing room, and I had been waiting and waiting for Sister's voice. I had intended to call back, 'Fabulous, I'm on my way,' or something of the sort, leap instantly to my feet, and get on with it. But I just sat there, shaking all over, suddenly aware of my heart thumping, my pulse rate going up, and feeling hot and cold.

'Come on, Sheila,' I heard Sister say again, in her cheerful voice, 'we're ready.' Somewhere behind me my friend Muriel said, 'Go on, Sheila, we're all with you.' I was thinking: 'This is what I've been waiting for, this should be the beginning of the great moment, at last ... or perhaps it won't be after all ...' I was terrified.

But I got to my feet, and then, instead of striding out the five yards or so, I walked slowly and haltingly. I could hardly make it at all. I got into the dressing room eventually, and hands guided me to the chair. I felt my way round it; an odd sort of chair for a hospital, I remember thinking in all the confusion of my mind – it was more like an office chair. It had arms that felt leathery, and a headrest. I sat in it, and gripped the arms as if my very life depended on hanging on. I squeezed the arms and my nails dug into the leather.

Then I could feel the bandages being unwound, and suddenly I did not want them to do it. Yet, at the same time, I couldn't do anything to stop them. I wanted to shout: 'Don't. Please don't do it.' Now that it had come, I just did not want to face the moment.

Then the bandages were off, and even then I did not know the result, because I had my eyes tight shut. I heard Sister saying, 'Come on, Sheila, open your eyes, the bandages are off ...' And I gripped the armrests even harder, and opened my eyes.

What happened then – the only way I can describe the sensation – is that I was suddenly hit, physically struck by brilliance, like an immense electric shock into my brain, and through my entire body. It flooded my whole being with a shock wave, this utterly unimaginable, incandescent brightness: there was white in front of me, a dazzling white that I could hardly bear to take in, and a vivid blue that I had never thought possible. It was fantastic, marvellous, incredible. It was like the beginning of the world.

Then I turned and looked the other way, and there were greens, lots and lots of different greens, different shades, all quite unbelievable, and at the same time with this brilliance there flooded in sound, the sound of voices saying, 'Can you see, can you see?' But I was just so overwhelmed and spellbound by the sensation that had occupied every bit of me, as if the sun itself had burst into my brain and body and scattered every molten particle of its light and colour, that it took me some time to say anything. I looked back at the blue and said, 'Oh it's blue, it's so beautiful.'

'It's me,' said Sister, coming towards me. The blue I could see was her uniform, and she came right up to me and touched me, and said, 'Sheila, can you see it?' But I was still not coherent, and turned away, and said, 'Green, it's wonderful.' And this was Annette, and Linda, and Ann, who had gathered round me, and said, 'It's us, it's our uniforms.'

Then they realised I could see properly, because there was something away to the left that appeared to me a sort of yellow colour. I did not know what it was, and said, 'What's that over there, that yellow thing?' And they said, 'It's a lamp, and it's really cream colour, pale cream.' But they knew for certain I could see it, though

I had not known it was a lamp, and I had got the colour wrong. My memory of colours was pretty murky, but I could still identify the strongest ones. But until that moment in my life I had no idea that there could possibly exist so many clear, washed colours.

All this, I know, took only a few seconds. Everything crowded in. Then, just as quickly, everything started to go misty and blurred. The colours began to fade, and merge into one another, and I thought, 'No, oh no, it's going. That's all there's going to be, I can't bear it ...' I was struck by a sudden terror, and put my hands instinctively up to my eyes – and found there were tears streaming down my face. I thought, 'Oh, thank goodness, it's not going, it's just the tears.' And I wept uncontrollably, and could not stop, because of the joy and the shock that I still could not fully take in, as, at the same time, everyone round me, Sister, nurses, and all sorts of people I did not know, were shaking my hand – and I could just see enough to realise that they, too, were crying, and could not say anything for tears.

The memory of those few seconds is indelible: the wonder, the sense of disbelief, yet belief, the sudden engulfing knowledge that I could see. I could see!

Then I had to have the bandages put back on again, but I did not care. I knew there was a flood of light outside, even if I had to be returned to the dark world where I had come from. And when the bandages were back on, I understood that before I had never really known the depth of that former permanent darkness, because the recollection of the first brief sight of brilliance remained in my mind, and the colours danced and merged still, and came and went in unending patterns, whirling away. As they did so, I was thinking, 'It's still so beautiful,' and I knew I had escaped from the infinite black pit.

I got back into the ward with steps shakier, if anything, than when I had left for the dressing room. I wanted to shout out at everyone there: 'I can see, I can see!' But what I managed was barely above a whisper. Everyone in the ward knew anyway. The news had gone before me, and I could feel how pleased everybody was for me, how overjoyed and overcome that it had happened, and this – the feeling that other people cared – was wonderful, too.

It was a strange realisation that all these people wished me well. It was like being surrounded by an embracing radiant warmth. I sat there in the ward in one of the armchairs, feeling this atmosphere all round me, and quite unable to take anything in. Here was something I had waited for; I had endlessly attempted to imagine what it might be like. But the reality was unlike anything that I had dreamed of. It was bewildering, and I could not fully comprehend all its meaning.

As I sat there, the thought was drumming away, 'I

must ring Don, I must tell him.' Then I heard Jasmine. She had guessed I would want to phone immediately, and because I was still crying, she said, 'Can I dial the number for you?' She had brought the mobile telephone already plugged in, and she added, 'Can I stand here while you tell him you can see?' I could feel her joy like a physical thing, and hear it in her voice.

But, however perfect you imagine things might be, they never are, and when I dialled the number myself, there was no reply from Don's surgery. He was out on his visits. I heard the number ringing and ringing, and thought, 'Do answer, I've got this to tell you, you must answer.' But the ringing tone went on and on, until I put the receiver down. Then I tried the number of his radio telephone service, so they could try his callsign, 269, and give him a message. It would not be the same as telling him myself, but he would get to know as soon as was possible.

I got through to this number immediately. 'I'd like you to give a message to 269.'

'Yes, certainly. What's the message?'

'Just tell him I can see.'

There was a pause, and the voice that came back had a very puzzled expression. 'Oh. Tell him that you can see?'

'Yes. Just tell him that.'

I put the phone down, feeling a bit deflated, because I really wanted to rush out of the hospital and wave all the traffic down on the road and tell them, or go and shout from the top of Everest, or go on to the radio worldwide and say, over and over, 'I can see, it's me, I can see …'

Instead, I rang my brother, and all I kept saying was, 'I can see, it's so marvellous, the colours are fabulous, and I never knew the world was so brilliant,' and then I rang practically every number I could think of, pouring coins into the box, and saying the same message. No one at the other end had much of a chance to say anything back, but I knew they were thrilled for me. I spent just over a pound in calls.

It was not until nearly midday that I heard from Don. He had received my message. He told me that he had been to see a patient, and got back to the car where Emma was sitting in the passenger seat waiting for him, and the call light of his radio telephone had come on. I suppose when he saw it he was nervous about answering, because he had been waiting all morning for a message; he sat there for a minute not daring to brace himself to the news, whether it would be infinitely good or heartbreakingly bad. He told me that when he did pick up the telephone and the message came through, he just had no reply. He sat in the driving seat unable to grasp the sheer wonder of the moment, and finally put his arms round Emma, and said, 'Emma, you'll never have to work again.'

·Later, when he came to see me that evening, we did not speak much at first. Neither of us could appreciate fully what had happened. We are so close, Don and I, that it was some time before we needed to put into words all the possibilities that were expanding in our minds, like a world suddenly starting to form, whirling round, taking shape, and getting bigger and bigger all the time.

Eventually all his sentences were beginning: 'When you come home ...' And each time there was something new he was going to show me. We sat and talked and planned there in the ward. He told me the leaves were turning from gold to red, and it meant something to me for the first time. He had built a new stone fireplace, and could not wait to show it to me. We would go on holiday ... life began to unfold in prospect, and now, instead of being bounded by the limits of my pool of blackness, it stretched on and out, full of light.

When Don had phoned earlier in the day, the nurses had been bringing the midday meal round. But I was too excited to eat. I kept thinking, 'If those colours were so beautiful, what about the rest, what about everything else?' The colours were still dancing and whirling about in my mind behind the bandages, changing pattern as in a child's kaleidoscope, and exploding like fireworks. What was it like outside? I wanted to tear the bandages off and rush to the window and see everything.

I also wanted Mr Shearing to come in. I kept thinking of his words, 'I don't work miracles, lassie.' But he had, and I wanted him to share all my feelings, and know how I thought about him, and everything else. I kept asking Sister, 'When will Mr Shearing be coming?' I knew he had not been able to be in the dressing room that morning because he had been operating. 'Oh, he'll be in as soon as he can,' she would reply. 'He's still in the operating theatre.' I sat there for most of that Monday afternoon, thinking, 'I do wish he would hurry up; I can't wait to tell him how marvellous it is,' and I kept wondering if he knew that the operation had worked beyond our wildest dreams.

Then, about four o'clock, I suddenly sensed a familiar smell in the distance. It was the faint aroma of cigar smoke. Mr Shearing! He was probably in with Sister, discussing what had gone on. Sure enough, I presently heard his familiar footsteps approaching along the ward, and I sat up. When the footsteps stopped, and I heard the voice say, 'Hello, lassie, how are you?' all my words suddenly tumbled out and rushed away with me in a great flood of emotion. 'Oh, it's so fantastic, it's wonderful, it's fabulous, oh, I can't tell you, it's marvellous ...' But his only comment was, 'Yes, isn't it marvellous Nottingham Forest won on Saturday.'

I was flabbergasted. I could hardly believe my ears. I said, 'Notts Forest? I don't care about Notts Forest. I can *see,* that's the marvellous thing.' He patted me awkwardly on the shoulder, and left. A minute or two later, Muriel came up, and said, 'I wish you could have seen his face. It looked as if it had been lit up. He just stood there, smiling at you.' And I realised that he had been at a loss for words. Gentle and humane person that he is, all the business about Nottingham Forest had just been a sidestep round something he was too moved to express.

So I was able to appreciate a little of his reaction, but it was not until I went back to the hospital a year later that I learned the full story of how Mr Shearing had really felt. At the hospital one of the other patients recognised me, and, by chance, her father had been in at the same time as I had originally, but in the men's ward upstairs. She told me, 'After Mr Shearing had been to see you, he went up to the men's ward, and went round telling everybody you could see, and how wonderful you thought it was, and how it really made him think that everything was worthwhile.' I then remembered sitting talking to him when he was telling me about the failures he had had in operations, and how terrible it was, and sad, that he had proved unable to do anything for these patients. I remember saying, 'But the successes must be worth everything.' He had agreed they were, and now I felt how tremendous it was that he had gone up to that ward and told everyone about it. He must have – or I certainly hope he must have – felt the immense joy of giving so much.

After Mr Shearing had gone, I waited for visiting time, and I was inundated with callers. Apart from Don, who had called every day, and my mother and father and Graham, none of my friends had been in up to then. But that evening I had about ten visitors all told. To every one of them I went on and on about what had happened during that two minutes in the dressing room. They just about got 'Hello' and 'Goodbye' in and handed me their presents of chocolates and flowers.

From that day, for the rest of the time in hospital, the bandages were taken off each morning for a couple of minutes, drops were put in my eyes, and clean bandages were put back. Apart from those two lucid, incandescent minutes, I inhabited my old world. But, increasingly, it became less and less like that familiar, enclosed world as I began to know more and more of what lay beyond. I was able to plan what I would look at each day during the brief seeing interval. I knew I would be struck each time by the blues and greens of uniforms, but I tried to consider what else I could take in quickly. All the same, every morning when the moment arrived for me to go to the dressing room, I had a flicker of doubt as I walked up the ward. I always thought, 'Will it be as bright again, will it be as beautiful?' Each morning it was, and the anxieties faded from my mind.

It was difficult to choose what to look at. One morning I took the bowl of dahlias in, the ones I had felt nothing for when they arrived. I also thought, 'I must remember to have a look at the colours of my dressing gown and my nightie.' Which might sound trivial, but it was important for me then. I wanted to know what I was wearing, and how I appeared. When I went down to the dressing room that morning I heard Sister say to me breezily, 'Whatever have you brought your flowers for, Sheila?' When I told her, she laughed, but it was good-natured laughter. When the bandages were removed, and I had got over the renewed shock of brilliance, I looked down at my dahlias and saw that they were a gorgeous yellow that I had never imagined, and that they seemed so intricately made. I was so fascinated by their every detail, and so remorseful that I had felt nothing for them, that I forgot to notice what I was wearing.

The following morning I did remember: my dressing gown was a wonderful turquoise, and my nightie purple. The combination sounds dreadful, but that did not occur to me at the time, particularly because on this occasion I had something of a shock. As I was looking down, I caught sight of my hands. I was appalled. They looked awful. I could not keep my eyes off them. I said to one of the nurses, 'Annette, look at my hands. Aren't they terrible.'

She came over, looked at them quite closely, and then said, 'What's terrible about them?'

'Well, look at them, look at the veins, and the knuckles. The bones stick out. Don't they look awful?'

'But they're perfectly normal.'

'They can't be.'

'But they are. Look at mine. Your hands are like everybody else's.'

So I looked at her hands, and saw the veins standing out, and said, 'Gosh, aren't they horrible things?' I always expected from the way that hands felt that they would look smooth and nice. I was really quite upset, and disillusioned. When Don came in that evening, I said to him, 'Look at my hands.'

'Yes. Well, they're all right. What's the matter?'

'But they're horrible.'

'No, they're not. They're beautiful hands.'

'But look at the veins standing out, and the knuckles. They're dreadful.'

'Of course they're not. Wait till you've seen mine. You'll see the veins and everything. Everybody's hands are like that.'

I really could not accept that my hands were at all like anyone else's. I went round for the next day or so, and until I got used to the idea, tucking them out of sight in my dressing gown sleeves.

The following day Mr Shearing came in again. He said that if I wanted I could go home the following day. It was like being given the order for release and pardon at last for a crime you have never committed. I rang Don immediately, I was so excited. That night was another sleepless one, waiting for Friday – the day when I would see the outside world for the first time, and really start my new life.

15

At First Sight

DON WAS DUE to pick me up at half-past twelve. All week he had been joking about having his hair dyed from grey to a different colour, and saying, 'It's all right for you, you know. I've seen you. I knew what you looked like to start with. But you've never seen me. You could be in for a shock.' I said, 'Whatever you look like, it won't make any difference.' It had never before crossed my mind to wonder what I might think of people's looks. I had no preconceived notion, in any exact sense, about how they might appear. Still further from my mind was the notion that from now on I would look at people, and what I saw would help to form my judgement of them, for better or worse, accurately or inaccurately, like the rest of the sighted world I was joining. It was a strange feeling.

I waited, wearing dark glasses which I had been given that morning. My eyes were still not accustomed to the general brilliance, and so had to be shaded for the time being. I walked up and down the ward, and still marvelled at the colours, dimmed as they were by the glasses. Even the very whiteness of the sheets and pillowcases on the beds impressed me. I looked at the bowls of flowers on the locker tops and thought to myself, 'I don't believe in evolution. Those flowers were always like that, perfect in every detail, but waiting for me to see them, specially made for me.' It was irrational, but that was the way I felt.

I sat by my bed, my cases packed, wondering what Don looked like – trying to imagine his face from the ideas I had received over the years. But it was no good. Then I heard the ward door open – it had a characteristic squeak – and heard Don's footsteps coming down the ward. I thought, 'Oh God, this is him. This is the moment,' and I looked up. I saw a stranger coming towards me, and did not for an instant connect him with Don. I thought fleetingly, 'Brown, suntanned, handsome,' and then, 'It's Don!' I could not grasp the idea properly, though. He was so much more distinguished-looking, and so very much more handsome than I could possibly have imagined. In one glance I took in his navy blue suit, very smart, and his tie that had little pink and yellow flowers on a blue background, and at the same time I was struck with the idea of how lucky I was to have a husband whom I not only loved already for everything I had not been able to see, but with whom I instantly fell in love all over again for his appearance.

He came up to me, and said, smiling, 'Hello, Petal.' My face told him, I am sure, all he needed to know about my reactions to his looks. I was grinning from ear to ear as I said, 'Hello.'

He picked up my cases and said, 'Well, come on then, come and have a look at the outside world. Emma's waiting in the car.' And I thought, 'Emma, dear Emma. I shall be seeing her for the first time as well. What a day!' I could not get out of the ward fast enough, with everyone waving and wishing me good luck. We went arm in arm through the doors and I said goodbye to Sister and the nurses. Then, when we reached the outer doors, it was like that first electric shock of sight all over again.

The sunshine burst in on me, and once more it was as I imagined the birth of the world. Of course I knew that it had been like this for millions and millions of years, or so my rational mind told me, but I still felt it was the entire Creation, suddenly laid on for my personal benefit. In the same thought was contained the idea that I was seeing for the first time something which everyone else was used to and took for granted, and its impression on me was unique.

Beyond the sunshine and immediate glaring radiance, I saw a great expanse of green.

'What's that?'

'Why, it's grass, of course.'

Grass? Of course. It had to be. Something I had felt through the soles of my shoes. 'But it's so green. I can't believe it. Is it always like this?'

Don said it was, but I had to kneel down and touch it to make sure it was what I had felt before, and it was.

'But it's all different shades, all different greens. Look at those patches. Even the separate blades seem to differ in colour.'

'Yes. It's always like that.'

'It's so marvellous, so beautiful.'

We went over towards the car, and Don went a bit ahead to let Emma out. The next thing I knew, she came bounding out of the car, and I could see the sun shining and glinting on her coat as she bounced up to me. I put my arms round her, and saw her tail going, making her whole body move, and her ears flapping. I cried, 'Oh, Don, isn't she *beautiful*.' People had told me she was brown, chocolate brown they had said, and that was the main impression I'd had of her appearance. I had also been told that she had a white patch on her chest, and her nose and eyes were brown, but none of it had really meant much to me. But now I could see her! No one had ever described her properly.

Her ears were a gingery colour. As the sun shone on them they were turned to a pale ginger. Her lovely

brown nose glistened. There was a gingery part along
her nose towards her eyes, and the auburn along her
back was rich and deep; it shaded off down her legs and
along her flanks into a soft brown. I have no way of
describing the effect she had on me except to say she
was more gorgeous than I could ever have imagined in
a thousand years. I said, 'Oh, Emma, you're so beautiful! Nobody ever told me. Everybody said you were
brown, but nobody told me you were a hundred shades
of brown.' Her reply was to wag her tail even more
vigorously, take one of the smaller bags from me, and go
rushing round with it on the grass. We had not been
together for ten days, and she was as thrilled to meet me
as I was to see her for the first time. She went off
towards the car holding the bag and dived into the back
seat with it, so making sure in her own mind that I was
not going to go away from her again. If she had the bag
it stood to reason that I would have to stay with her!

I got in, and Emma kept touching me with her nose,
while I stroked her affectionate head. It was odd
sitting in the car that I had been in so many times, but
about the appearance of which I had no idea, from the
dashboard to the upholstery. It was odd, too, watching
Don driving, changing gear, steering. I had never
thought about it, and had barely appreciated that so
much was involved. I kept looking at him, and
thinking, 'Isn't he good-looking? Isn't he fabulous?

Aren't I lucky?' He looked at me from time to time, not saying much at all.

Once out of the hospital gates I began to look out of the car more, and all sorts of things came tumbling in on my consciousness. 'Those orange lines down there, what are they for?'

'Oh, they're double yellow lines – there are single yellow lines as well. They tell you where you can park and where you can't.'

'When did they put them there?'

'They've been there for years.'

'Are you sure?'

'Mm … they've been there for ages.'

It was slightly unnerving seeing things the existence of which I had never even suspected. 'Don, look. There are all sorts of white lines along the road.'

'Yes. They've been there even longer.'

I thought, 'I suppose no one would ever have dreamt of telling me that there were white and yellow lines on the roads; they wouldn't have thought I'd be interested.' Seeing them, I was fascinated. The verges, too. I had no idea they were all so grassy, or that there were so many trees.

'Don, look at the trees. Are there always as many as this?'

'Yes. They're all over the place, thousands of them. Even in the city.'

Of course I knew there were trees. I'd always been aware of them, and could hear them when the wind blew. But I had never imagined so many, or that they were everywhere, growing out of pavements, in gardens, and, as we drove through the countryside towards Nottingham, more and more of them, all different shapes. I could not get over the shapes, some round, some tall, and all in varying, breathtaking shades of green.

Don said, 'All trees are like that. Even the same kind of tree – oak, beech, chestnut, or whatever – can vary in shape when you look at it.' And I looked and looked at them as we drove along, with the sun catching them and somehow becoming entangled in the branches and leaves, and throwing moving shadows, so that the trees looked as if they were made in layers, like frills. I could see the leaves being moved by the wind, and said, 'They look as if they're doing a dance in the wind.'

All the people intrigued me, and I am sure that Don, kind as he is, must have wanted to laugh at me. 'Gosh,' I said, 'look at all the people on the pavement. They've all got different coloured clothes. It's fantastic.' But Don did not laugh. He just said, 'Yes, when you've been in the car before, you won't have realised they were there, because you couldn't hear them once you were on the move.' He was right. I had known there were countless people all around, but when you can't see, a car insulates you; you don't think about all the human beings outside it doing their shopping, or going to work, or going to the pub, or standing talking.

I kept saying to Don, 'Look at the houses, they're all different, they've all got different coloured doors.' Yellow lines, white lines, posters, buses, road signs, shops ... it was like a journey to somewhere you had never been before, somewhere you had never thought existed, a new world, all rotating past the car window like an enormous merry-go-round.

When we were nearly home I remembered my flowers. I had so many beautiful bouquets, and bunches of roses, dahlias and freesias that even the hospital had more than enough for other patients, and had said they did not mind my taking some home. But in the excitement the flowers had quite gone out of my mind. I was rather upset, at the thought of all the people who had sent them or brought them being, so to speak, casually neglected, rebuffed even. 'Can't we go back?' I asked Don, but he said, 'Oh, it's a terribly long way, and we're nearly home now. It doesn't matter.' But it did matter. Another thought pushed this one aside. My Siamese cats had been boarded out. Pat, a good friend who herself bred Siamese, had taken Ming with her four-week-old kitten. Sandra had taken Hera, my Red Point and her litter of four, and yet another friend had taken my male Lilac Point. I was dying to see them all, and, now I knew that colours were nothing like I had imagined, to find out what they were really like. 'Oh Don,' I said, 'are the cats all right? Can we fetch them back this afternoon?' But he just said, 'Now, don't worry about the cats. Everything's sorted out. You just come home, and everything will be fine.' By this time we were in the road where we lived. It all looked more lovely than I'd imagined, with the trees and the roses in people's front gardens. Then we drew up at the gate. I got out, and Emma leaped over the seat, and got in front of me, tail wagging. As we opened the door, Emma rushed in first, and went straight to fetch me various gifts to show how pleased she was that I was home.

I walked into the living room, my living room, and saw it for the first time. Like so much else, it was different from my mental image: because so much had been dark and dismal in my mind, I hadn't pictured what a lovely room it was. I was delighted. I suddenly thought that Don had had the rich red carpet specially put down for me, but when I knelt down and touched it, I realised he hadn't. It was the same carpet we had always had. Then he said, 'What do you think of the fireplace?' This was lovely, all the stone he had carefully laid, with fawns and pinks, and throwing shadows where they jutted out. I noticed the horse brasses that I had cleaned every week, and saw their sparkle for the first time.

Then I suddenly caught sight of the biggest bouquet of flowers imaginable in the middle of the table – pinks, roses, dahlias, all overflowing the bowl and dominating the room. 'Don,' I said, 'you shouldn't have. They're wonderful. What a homecoming! No wonder you didn't mind about the hospital flowers!'

So much for my anxiety in the car. In the next instant, my other small worry was dispelled. I realised, turning away from the flowers, and with quite a start, that there was someone else in the room. I caught a movement in the corner of my eye, looked round, and saw a woman standing over by the window. I had no idea who it was.

'Who's that?' I said, staring at her, and having not a glimmer of recognition (whose face, on reflection, could I have recognised immediately?). She started to laugh, but would not say anything, and I racked my brains trying to think who it was. Then she said, still laughing, 'It's me.' Instantly I knew the voice. 'Pat,' I said, 'what are you doing here?'

'Well, I've brought your cats.'

'You mean Ming and the kitten. How marvellous.'

'No, not just Ming and the kitten. I've got all the rest as well. I thought you'd want to see them all as soon as you could.'

Pat disappeared into the kitchen, and, a second later, round the door came Ming. What struck me immediately was how intensely blue her eyes were, and, as I took in her other details – her shining black face, her paws, her ears – I reacted in the same way as when, only an hour before, I had seen Emma for the first time. With Ming, and with my other cats as they came in later, I was not at all prepared for the variety of colours and shades that no one and no textbook had ever told me about. I had originally chosen to have Siamese because they were so smooth and svelte, but to see them was a revelation, and the greatest pleasure of all was to watch them move. It was as if they floated over the ground.

Eventually Don had to go back to the surgery, and do his round of patients, and Pat had to leave, too. This left me in the house on my own (apart from the animals) and I quite liked the idea, because it gave me an opportunity to look round at everything I wanted to see. I sat on the settee, with Emma next to me, and I looked at her. Don had often said that Emma had an old-fashioned look, and I saw the expression he meant when we sat there on that first afternoon: a look that suggested great moral virtue. I smiled at her, putting out my hand to stroke her. She put her head forward towards my hand, and I thought, 'I wonder if she's been doing that for the past ten years when I put out my hand, not knowing exactly where she was?'

It was so marvellous to sit and look at Emma (even more than a year later I have still not got over my fascination as I look at people and animals) and watch her face change to a kind of delight, with her ears going up, and the end of her tail brushing the carpet. As we sat there, I thought of all the things I wanted to do, now I was home.

One of the first items was to look into a mirror. I had seen Don, Emma, Ming and the other cats. But I had not yet seen myself! I could have done in hospital, I suppose, but I hadn't wanted to. I wanted to save this most personal experience until I was on my own, for I was more than a little apprehensive. I had no idea what to expect. One half of my mind prompted, 'Come on, get it over with. It's got to be done, and waiting won't alter the result for better or worse.' The other half of my mind insisted on delaying. I suppose I sat on the settee for nearly a quarter of an hour, stroking Emma, and summoning up the will to go and do what had to be done.

When I could not see, I had never really thought much about the existence of mirrors, and the house, naturally, was not over-endowed with them. I supposed there was one in the bathroom for Don to see himself shaving. While I was sitting there, turning these thoughts over in my mind, I was looking round the room again. Apart from mirrors, I had never thought very much about the existence of the pictures on the wall, either. I had known they were there, but the objects that blind people do not come into contact with constantly by touch are not retained in the forefront of the mind. At least, that was my experience. Don used to paint in his spare time, and there were some of his canvases on the wall. I found them intriguing, and remember looking at them, and trying consciously to sort out which was which from memory.

One that he had done was a copy of Rembrandt's *Man in the Golden Helmet*. I was fascinated by the gold, and the intricate work on the helmet. To the left, I recalled, there was a seascape. When I went to look at this, I encountered for the first time the difficulty which was to crop up quite frequently in those first few days out of hospital. This was the problem of relating the reality of the image transmitted through the eyes to the brain, to a previous reality which was conditioned by touch or verbal description. Some objects that I saw for the first time I could identify immediately, although I still do not know why. But with others I had not the least notion of what they might be, until I felt them. The seascape I could make no sense of whatsoever. When Don brought me a cup of tea the following morning, I looked at the cup and had no idea what it was until I touched it.

But, back to looking into the mirror. At last, after examining our various pictures, and sitting with Emma, I made a move to the bathroom, and there confronted myself. I saw, as with Don coming up the ward, but even more unnerving, a total stranger. I did not know what to think. The lips moved when I moved mine, and the eyes blinked when I blinked. Seemingly these were the only points of contact between me and the looking glass image. Looking back, I suppose I should not have expected sudden recognition. How could I suddenly form an opinion of myself? Of my hair I thought, 'Not bad, not bad, it's really just about the same colour as Emma's.' The feature I kept on looking at was my nose. I put my hand up to touch it, because I could not believe it. I felt it, and it felt as it always had done. It hadn't grown. But to see it was an awful shock. It looked grotesque and clown-like; it dominated my entire face. Why had no one told me about my nose? Don, my mother, all my friends, must have known about it all along and kept quiet out of politeness. I was so upset, I could not look any longer. I felt miserable that I had a nose that stuck out so far, and it took me a long time before I was reassured that it was not extraordinary.

To get away from the thought of my nose I went into the bedroom, and looked into the wardrobe at all the clothes which friends had helped me buy, or which I had bought myself after having them described to me by the assistant in the shop. Some were awful. There were colours that did not go with one another, and others that were far too bright and gaudy for my liking. I was quite taken with some dresses I hadn't previously liked:

the texture of the material had not pleased me and I was surprised to find they were very pretty. It was a strange sensation – these were the outfits I had worn, all unknowing. But now the exciting thing was the prospect of being able to go out and choose my own clothes and start a fresh wardrobe. That cheered me up, nose or no nose.

I went back into the sitting room and sat down, and looked round me once more. I loved the curtains, and the carpet, and the wallpaper. Everything was so colourful, and looked to me fresh and new. I had lived here for years, but it was like being in a different home. It was not the home of my imagination at all, but a brighter, more spacious, more comfortable place altogether.

By this time, I was getting rather hungry, particularly since I had not had anything at lunchtime. I would have to go out to the shops and buy something for tea. I was itching to do this, in fact, to go out on my own. What would it be like? The shops were not far away, on the corner, and I knew them well. I wanted to see them. I found my shopping bag in the hall, and got to the front door, with Emma sensing we were about to go for an outing, and getting excited. But at the door I stopped. Exactly how would I do it? I felt instantly apprehensive. My original idea had been that I would go with Emma on the lead. But now I decided that for this first time I had better put on her harness, and let her take me along. Then, when I was thoroughly used to going out, we could dispense with the harness.

I picked the harness off the peg and Emma immediately went wild. She bounced up and down, and barked, and shook herself, and was overjoyed that after all this time of separation we were at last going out together again. It would be like old times for her, though not for me. I asked Emma to find the shops, and she took me out of the gate and along the footpath. But as soon as we were on our way, I suddenly saw the pavement rushing by under me. It was so unexpected and frightening, that I had to tell Emma to stop. In a moment I recovered and we went on again. But then I saw the fence coming at us at a headlong rate, and the trees seeming to fly towards us as if they were going to knock us down. Looking down again, I saw the pavement and even the shadows of the lamp posts were sweeping along towards me like solid black bars, making me think I would trip. It was no good. Once more I had to tell Emma to stop. I knew it was illogical. I knew I was moving, and not the lamp posts, or the pavement, or the shadows. But as far as I was concerned visually, the reverse was happening. I decided to give it another try. The same thing happened again. I was panic-stricken. I had to keep stopping to reassure myself that it really was me in motion, and each time we stopped Emma sat down and looked at me with those great brown eyes full of questions. She wanted to know what was happening; after ten years together why was I behaving in this peculiar fashion? In the end the only solution I could think of was to close my eyes, and let Emma carry on as usual. And this is how we finally arrived at the shops.

Emma stopped. I opened my eyes, and there we were, outside the greengrocer's. Immediately I was hit by a mass of colour, and that, mixed with some relief at actually being there, made me think, 'Well it was worth it after all.' I was astounded at the sight of all the fruit and vegetables and flowers in the window, and saw to my immense surprise that each apple in its redness or greenness was different, and that no two potatoes looked alike, nor the lettuces, nor anything in the whole array. How could there be so many shades and varieties of colour?

Apart from this, there were a lot of things in the window that I could not identify at all. Once again I was coming up against the problem of not being able to relate my previous tactile impressions to my present vision. Perhaps I had already that day given my brain enough to cope with. Seeing was miraculous, but I had, in a way, to learn to see as well. In the shop, where they knew me very well and were delighted at the success of my operation, they didn't mind my touching things I could not recognise. There was something on the counter that I could not, try as I would, put a name to. I could see some red, and green, and a shape. That was all it meant to me. It would not fit any description I could think of. Then I touched it. I realised I was seeing leaves and flowers. It was a plant. I could not understand why I had not immediately known what it was. It turned out to be a poinsettia. Then I pointed to something on the shelf, and said, 'What's that?' 'Celery.' 'And those?' 'Beetroot,' they said. So I went on, and finished up buying tomatoes because they looked the most gorgeous colour of all.

On our way back, I determined to keep my eyes open, which led to an odd incident. I was again in a state of nerves, but resolving to persevere, when I saw a young lad coming towards us. As usual, I was talking to Emma as we walked, and I said, 'Now there's someone coming, Emma, do be careful.' What she made of that unnecessary comment, I have no idea, but as I said it, I thought, 'Now I must take action, I must get round this boy. But how? How do I do it?' It did not occur to me that I was abandoning my trust and faith in Emma. I thought, 'I'll step aside to the right, and we'll avoid him that way.' So, when he was nearly up to us, I stepped to the side of the pavement to go right. In the very same second, Emma had decided the best way to take us past the lad was to go left. I let go of the harness, and we landed up in a sort of confused heap and a tangle of harness – while the lad went merrily on, all unaware. I felt dreadful, and I knew by Emma's expression she could not make out what had happened. She yawned, not out of boredom, but embarrassment.

She sat looking at me with an anxious, quizzical expression, which said, 'Why ever did you do that? In ten years you've never done that before. What's happened?' I said, 'Oh, Emma, I'm sorry, I shouldn't have put your harness on.' I decided that I had been expecting too much of her. I had virtually been asking her to stand by me until I had the courage to go out on my own. It was not fair. From then on, whenever we went out, I would simply have to put her on a lead, and learn how to manage myself.

We somehow got home from the shops, and then I took great delight in being able to empty my shopping bag and see to prepare a meal. But one thing I was already beginning to realise was that it took a great deal of concentration to look at objects. It was something quite new to me, this concentration and mental effort involved with seeing, something I had not suspected would be required. I had imagined that once I got my sight back, I would be able to see, and that would be that. But it was not the case. It was like suddenly being given an extra limb, and having to work hard at getting used to putting it to the best advantage. But it was exciting, too.

When I looked into the food cupboard for the first time, I found an Aladdin's cave full of tins and packets and jars which I did not know by sight, but which I had used before. They had taken on a new existence. I came across a packet that was red, yellow and white, and thought, 'What's this?' Of course, it said SALT on it, but, although years before I had been able to read print, regaining this faculty took a long time, and the word SALT at first was just an arrangement of different shaped letters. I could remember some printed words in my mind, and was able to write them down when I could not see. But, the other way round, presented with words via my eyes, and required by the brain to attach a meaning to them, was something altogether different, and very difficult at first, though it came back in time.

So, to begin with, I identified the salt by the old method, taste, and related this to the colour of the box. Cereal packets were yellow, or white with a pattern on them, baked bean tins were a distinctive turquoise blue, and so on.

Still, this was all discovery, and I did not mind. In fact I enjoyed going through the food cupboard on that first afternoon, and I enjoyed even more the preparation of the meal, with all the reds and greens of the salad dazzling me, even down to the simple business of running water from the tap over the lettuce: the way the water glistened and swirled, caught the light, and made a waterfall pattern in the sink fascinated me. Once I had laid the tea table, and was waiting for Don to come home, I went out into the garden, my lovely garden. I was so proud of it as I walked about, with Emma rooting along beside me.

When I was blind, there had been times when I literally hated those trees in the garden, because the branches were always getting tangled up in my hair, and if ever I did take a walk round the lawn, which was a fairly rare occurrence, I used to have to keep in mind the presence and arrangement of the three apple trees, and make sure I did not collide with them. The apple trees, in fact, had been nothing more than rather ogre-like obstacles, to be avoided and shunned. Now they not only looked incapable of harm, but beautiful, too. And at the edge of the grass was our willow tree. I could not get over its sheer grace. The leaves were green on one side, and silver on the other. For a moment I thought my eyes really had got it wrong. No one had ever told me that trees could have silver leaves. It was while I was looking at the willow that I noticed the sky for the first time, and how the clouds moved, sailing along, with great billows of white on blue. I heard the car draw up, and the gate latch click. Don was back.

He came up and joined me on the lawn, and said, 'Hello, how have you been getting on? What have you been doing?'

'Oh, looking at everything, you know.'

'What are you looking at now?'

'Well, to tell you the truth, I'm waiting to see the sunset.'

Don had often described the sunset to me and no one could have done it better, or more vividly, yet, standing there with him in the garden as the sun was going down, and the colours were just beginning to change in fractions of a second, I knew that there was no substitute for sight. Reading about things, or having them described (and I do not want to devalue in any way what Don had done) were substitutes, and until that day all I had ever had were second-hand sunsets.

On this Friday we stood and watched together. The sun disappeared, and the clouds and sky around were streaked with gold and purple. It was perfect, and to end that day nothing could have matched it.

16

A New Life

FOR THE FIRST few seconds after I woke up the following morning, everything seemed normal. It was no different from any other morning, from the ten thousand other times I had woken up. In front of me was a familiar blank greyish mist. Then I remembered. I could see! I had only to open my eyes, and I could see! It was the first morning of a new life. But, in my drowsiness, I wondered: 'Is it all really true? Dare I open my eyes?'

The night before, tired as I was, I had not wanted to go to sleep. It had seemed such a waste to spend eight hours with my eyes shut. I had lain there feeling happier than I had ever felt in my life before. Emma had got into her basket at the foot of the bed, and I had looked at the wallpaper, unable to keep my eyes off it. It was so pretty, with cascades of blossom on a deep rose background. Don had got into bed beside me, and I remember him saying, 'We can go anywhere we want, you know.' I really did think that the world, at last, was mine. But I was still looking at the wallpaper when we put the light out.

Now I opened my eyes. Immediately I saw that the wallpaper was still there. I could read, I could take Emma for walks, I could see everything I had heard about and been told about, and never properly known. An astronomer who sees a new planet must, I thought, feel like this, or an explorer coming to the edge of a plateau and seeing below him miles and miles of unexplored territory. As I lay daydreaming, the sun was streaming through the curtains, and I saw Emma still curled up in her basket.

Then Don stirred and said he would get up and make some tea, which brought me back to the more immediate, practical things of life. And while I was looking at Emma, she woke too. She got out of her basket, stretched sleepily right down on her forelegs with eyes half-closed against the brightness of the day, but looking up at me, full of affection. She gave her usual brisk and vigorous good morning shake, then, wagging her tail jumped up on the bed. I had heard all this every day, but never before seen what happened. It was a daily ritual that she had to play her game of what Don calls 'Push Noses' in which she puts her nose under the bedclothes and pushes – back legs in the air and tail waving frantically. Actually seeing this for the first time, accompanied by the normal sounds, I lay back and shook with laughter, it was so funny.

At that moment Don came in with the tea, and I said to him, 'I wonder how long it will be before she realises I can see?' Emma had obviously not yet grasped the fact, and I wondered whether it would dawn on her gradually or suddenly. Then something odd happened. I was watching Don pour out the tea and start to get dressed, when I noticed his legs. I hadn't noticed them before he got into bed the night before, and I looked, and said, 'Don, your legs.'

'What about my legs?'

'Aren't they strange?' And I started to giggle because they looked so peculiar to me.

Poor Don was quite put out. He looked down and, with a great muster of dignity, said, 'They're perfectly normal legs.'

'But they can't be.'

'Yes, they are.'

'But they're all wrong somehow. They don't seem to fit the rest of your body.'

He then turned round and hurriedly put on his trousers to cover his legs and hide them from my critical gaze: I was convinced they were out of proportion. I have no idea how I expected legs to look, but whatever image I had it was not matched by Don's lower limbs. When I got out of bed a second or two later, I stopped laughing. I saw that my legs looked peculiar as well, amazingly strange, and disproportionate.

Over breakfast, I discovered something else. I cooked bacon and eggs and tomatoes. I thought how much pleasure I had missed by not being able to see food, and how the sight of it added to the appetite. We sat down, and I put my fork towards the bacon, and, somehow, the two did not connect. I could see the bacon, and I could see the prongs of the fork near it, but I could not bring the two together. The coordination was beyond me, and although it was an admission of a temporary setback, an unforeseen defeat even, I had to revert to my old ways and feel for my food with my knife and fork. I stopped concentrating on looking, and went back to touch.

Over the coffee, Don said, 'Where would you like to go today?' He had arranged to have a week off from the surgery, and was longing to take me on all sorts of trips in the car. Before he said it I knew where I wanted to go first: 'What about Newstead Abbey, what about going there?' Newstead Abbey, with its acres of woods, lakes and gardens is about a twenty-minute drive out of Nottingham on the Mansfield side. Once it was the home of Lord Byron, and in the 1930s was presented to Nottingham City Corporation. I had been there so many times when I was blind, and I found it always so peaceful. I could almost feel the atmosphere of the old abbey, and would imagine Byron writing poetry under the trees, or riding his horse along the paths. I used to go round and feel the trees, knowing there were great masses of rhododendrons, and hear the waterfalls. I was dying to see it all.

There was a lake which stretched like a great looking glass, with moorhens and swans floating on it, attached to their shimmering mirror images. Eventually we came to the waterfalls. The sun was shining, and it caught the water, and turned it into a cascade of diamonds, whirling and dancing over the stones. The colours were changing in a halo over the falls. I could not take my eyes off it, and Don almost had to drag me to look at the flowers he had caught sight of: dahlias and chrysanthemums in a blaze of different yellows and bronzes and scarlets. To me it was as if all the colour in the world had suddenly been concentrated and massed in that spot. Then I caught sight of a stone wall, a part of the old abbey, and went over to see it. It was mottled all over with pinks, whites, yellow, grey, brown, with mosses and lichen growing in the crevices, and all made up of a million tiny details.

I felt quite high on colour and visual sensations. But one last thing I had to see. That was Byron's memorial to his Newfoundland dog, Boatswain. We reached the little square stone edifice at the top of some steps. Emma went all round it, very interested. And I was able, at last, to read for myself what Byron had written about his dog. Inscribed on the stone it said that Boatswain possessed 'Beauty without Vanity, Courage without Ferocity, and all the Virtues of Man without his Vices.' I wished that I had written that. But in praise of Emma.

Every day we went out somewhere different, and every morning I went into the garden to look at things. One morning, as we were waiting to go out, I called to Don, 'Come and have a look at this bird.'

He came rushing out of the house, probably thinking that something strange was happening.

'Look,' I said, 'at the bird sitting in that tree.'

'Yes,' he said, puzzled, 'what's the matter with it?'

'No, there's nothing the matter with it, but look, it's sitting there in the branches.'

'Yes,' he said patiently, 'I can see.'

He did not get the point of my excitement, nor should I have expected him to. I had to explain. I had known, because I had either been told, or read it, that birds sit in trees. I had always been aware of birds around me, above me somewhere. I could even tell the difference between some birds. I knew blackbirds' calls and sparrows' chirpings. But my mind had never been able to connect the idea of the birds with the idea of trees. I could never put them together, somehow. It sounds mad, but it was so. Despite having been told, my brain could not make the link. And here I was actually *seeing* a bird in a tree.

On the last morning of our holiday, Don had a brilliant idea. 'What about going up to Yorkshire, to Flamborough Head, say?' I knew that up there it was supposed to be very beautiful, and I could not wait to get in the car and start. I was longing for my first view of the sea.

It was a long drive, almost a hundred miles, and on the way countryside rolled by, through the Dukeries, beyond the coalfields and industrial towns, and gradually into the wide, green and steep hills of the Yorkshire Wolds. The fields rolled away ahead and on either side. Sometimes we would be going past a church in a dip, at the next moment we were at the top, looking over undulating greenness. I remembered learning about contours in geography, but I had never before seen what they really meant.

Don drove the car up to the lighthouse at Flamborough Head, with its brilliant white tower, and we got out, Emma running ahead. A second or so after hearing a great booming and roaring, I saw the sea. I had never imagined such endless movement, such brilliance, such force of motion. The sea seemed to gather strength, pausing for a moment of silence, then it came roaring in, dashing and thundering against the foot of the cliffs, while in the circle formed by the coast, the water appeared to boil. The first time this happened, I caught hold of Don's arm. I felt sure the cliff was trembling and would crumble under the assault. But when the wave retreated from the worn foot of the cliff, I realised that this had been happening for centuries, and that I was quite safe. Emma loved Flamborough too. She ran about, and helped us when eventually we went down to the beach to collect some pebbles and shells. She dashed in and out of the sea, shaking herself with happiness. I picked up all sorts of different stones from the beach, and we took them home as a memento.

But, among all the tumbling impressions of that week, there was a touch of sadness, too. I had time to go through all the drawers and cupboards, and I came across old letters, forgotten books and magazines, and photographs. It was looking at the photographs especially that brought home to me that there were some things I did not know about when I was blind, and would almost have preferred to keep that way. There were pictures of my family, and I saw that they seemed older than I had imagined them. I found snaps of Ohpas, my Siamese cat who had died, and wished I had not come across them. Above all, there were a whole lot of photographs of Emma, all lovely, from the age of a few weeks, some of them sent to me by Paddy Wansborough, and showing what a gorgeous, lively little puppy she must have been. Others showed her later in the fullness of her vigour and looks, and continued up to the present. The trouble was that, looking at them one after the other, I could see the process of Emma's growing up and getting older. I knew she was nearly eleven, but I never thought of her as that old. Her age did not mean anything to me until I saw those photographs, and then it suddenly hit me, even though she still looked her lovely self, with not a grey hair. I was confronted all at once with the fact that, for a dog, Emma was getting on.

And sadness was not the only unpleasant sensation. During the week, I went one afternoon to do some shopping in Nottingham, and this brought the most terrifying demonstration of how I had to learn to use my sight: any expectation I might have had that the possession of sight would automatically make life easy was very painfully revised. I got off the bus, and went out of the bus station. To say I was shocked would be nowhere near the truth. I was, all at once, scared out of my wits. I was with Emma on the lead, and as we emerged, added to all the noise and sense of bustle I knew about and had expected, there was revealed the cause: people, thousands of people, everything on the move, and cars and buses and cyclists going past and all mingled in a great melee. I could not believe there could be so many people, and not one of them took any particular notice of Emma and me. Why should they have done? I was no longer blind and Emma was not wearing a guide dog's harness. I had always relied on Emma implicitly to take me through crowds and people, but now I was bumped and jostled, and I realised that I was making no effort to get out of the way.

It was frightening, but we carried on, and then I happened to look up and see an enormously tall office building, part of the new centre of Nottingham. I had never thought anything could be so towering, or so threatening. It seemed to sway. I knew the clouds were going past above, but it looked as if the buildings were moving and not the sky. Feeling dizzy, I finally managed to look away and get back to the business of dividing everything into moving and non-moving obstacles, just as Emma had done for me all those years. Emma, of course, trotted along, and although she was still not used to being out with me, particularly in town, without her harness, she was very much like any other dog out for a walk on the lead. For most of the time that is. But there came a moment when she sensed I was in difficulties, and she reverted immediately and absolutely to the role she knew best. We were going over a crossing controlled by traffic lights. I waited for the green light, and, just as important, listened for the bleeping and the traffic stopping, because I still relied on hearing a great deal; half-way across the road I was aware that there was something in our path. I had no idea what it was; I could not work it out. The image was there, but my brain would not translate for me. I stood with Emma in the middle of the crossing in front of this object. Then Emma came to the rescue. From walking to heel, she came out in front of me and started pulling left on the lead. I followed. She took me down the middle of the road, then across to the opposite pavement. When I turned and looked back at the crossing I saw the bewildering object from a different angle, and realised what it was: one of those very long, flat trailers. It was empty, and had stopped, straddled over the crossing.

On the bus that took me home I was able to see at first hand all manner of differences in the passengers, and it was a continuing source of amazement: some happy, others miserable looking; some I thought I would like to know, but a lot more I would have run a mile from. All in all, I was disappointed by people's appearances. If they had had a uniformity in my blind thoughts, at least they shared a certain imagined handsomeness, and I had never allowed for human beings looking ugly, grotesque, even repulsive. In front of me sat a man whose neck bulged and rolled over his collar, and further down the bus was a bald man. Baldness, in particular, horrified me then, although by now I have become used to it.

Of course I was particularly surprised at how different my family and friends looked from what I had imagined. When I answered the door one day and saw a man standing there (it was before I had seen the family photographs) I had no idea until he spoke that it was my brother, Graham. And when my mother came round, I looked at her, and said, 'My goodness, haven't you gone grey? When did that happen?' I was tactless and possibly unkind in these encounters without meaning to be. It was only the surprise of reality that made me so.

I took some time also to get used to the idea of facial expressions. I looked at Don from time to time, and thought: 'People don't have one face, they have hundreds.' In a blind world there is only one hazy idea of what a face might be. There is no thought for that face being capable of change through laughter, sadness, or any other expression. And my face, too, was changing. During that first week our friends Eddy and Mike Blain came round, and after they had been with us about half an hour, Mike said, 'You've changed.'

'Whatever do you mean?'

'Well, your face has changed.'

'My face? How?'

'I don't really know. But it's different ... I don't know, I suppose it looks somehow more alive, Sheila. You're using expression.'

And it suddenly came to me that he must be right, and that the slight stiffness I had begun to feel in my face was nothing to do with the operation, as I had thought; instead it was caused by using facial muscles I had never used before. I suppose that children pick up expressions from their parents and from other children. But, never having seen a face well enough to mimic, I was now making up for lost time. I was glad Mike had told me that my face had become alive.

Before the operation, when I went out with Don, either to friends or to the pub for a drink, I would be with him, yet among a lot of people, and, unless he was talking directly to me or I could hear him, I would feel that the circuit between us had somehow been switched off. After I could see, it was marvellous to be able to look across a room full of people and see him instantly, and, no matter how many people were around, smile and see him smile back.

The time came all too quickly for Don, after that wonderful week, to go back to the surgery. Eventually I, too, went back to work. Emma was a little more used to being on the lead, but it must have been strange for her going on the familiar morning journey into Nottingham without having to take charge. She was still a bit puzzled, and looked at me occasionally before we were going out as if she were wondering: 'Where's my harness? I don't understand.' When we got to work, we went up to the door, and momentarily, I thought: 'I suppose this is the right place, but the door looks strange.' It was as if I had never known it. Yet as soon as I touched the handle, I knew it was the right place.

Inside, too, it was like somewhere I had never known, utterly different from the idea I had built up. When I reached the switchboard I had worked at for so long, I could hardly believe my eyes. My braille machine was there still, ready for use. I hadn't thought of braille in the past few weeks. I felt as if I were an archaeologist discovering a long-hidden relic of my own past. Emma did not seem to mind though. She went into her basket and settled down straight away.

At first I couldn't manage the new way. It was too much to operate the switchboard visually. I learned in time, but at the beginning I reverted to working it as I had always done, by touch. Similarly, it was difficult to write messages instead of using the braille machine. At home, I had started to teach myself to read again, and to write. But it came slowly. Once again, my brain would not always immediately attach the correct meanings to the shapes I saw on paper. Nevertheless, however hard it was, nothing could diminish the sheer pleasure of being given back the ability to read, and I spent my time surrounded by books and magazines.

I went on working at the garage for some time, until, in fact, I decided to start writing this book. As time went on, I gradually managed to operate the switchboard visually, and to write down all my messages, and, as happens quite quickly in life, old and familiar habits and patterns, once shed, were soon forgotten. I was reminded of my former way of life quite dramatically, and painfully, when the question arose of training my replacement. This was to be my friend Kath, with her guide dog Rachel bringing her to work. I had to train her on the switchboard, and doing this, and seeing her work, was like seeing myself as a ghost.

It was such a strange feeling, I could not believe that I had once been like that. But it came back to me in all sorts of ways. Kath felt my pen and pad, and laughed. 'They're no good to me,' she said. And I remembered how I used to feel: not wanting to admit that such things existed, things that I could not use. All the same, it had its amusing side. Rachel and Emma had to share the same dog bed, at least they tried, although it was rather a squeeze. Poor Emma kept getting out and looking up at me appealingly, and I interpreted this as meaning something like: 'Look, what's happening? I know I rather like Rachel, but I've been here so many years, and now she wants to come and take over my basket!' In the end she was so put out that she settled for lying by my feet on the carpet, despite all my explanations to her.

But the training was no laughing matter to me. I had to remember how to work the switchboard by touch, and train Kath to do so, and when she first sat down I had to demonstrate its workings by touch, her hand following mine over the braille indicators, feeling where all the numbers and switches were. I had to teach her where the braille lists were kept, and as I was doing this, in a terrible flash I suddenly knew how sighted people reacted to blind people. I knew how people must have looked at me. And yet, even now, with my experience, I still did not know how best to help Kath.

I kept wanting to tell her how to do something quicker because I could see it. Someone would ring the switchboard, and instantly I could see what was happening, and what number it was, but at the same time I could see Kath running her hands along the switchboard, feeling for the movement of the indicator to answer the call. I was so frustrated by this I wanted to say to her, 'No, you're on the wrong side, it's over the other side, it's the one at the top.' But I knew I would not be helping her if I did. It was heart-rending, and nothing else since leaving hospital has moved me so much. It hurt particularly because Kath was such a capable blind person, and such a good friend, and I could hardly bear it when she looked at people and could not see them, or I saw her feeling round her desk for her tea.

But life went on. Emma realised in time that I could see, and this happened, as I thought it might, as a result of one special incident. She was still in the habit of patiently waiting for the cats to finish their food every evening, and, having perfected a method of stealing across the kitchen floor without me hearing her, of going and polishing off what was left. The first I would know about it was always the rattle of empty feeding bowls, which was too late for anything to be done. One particular evening, however, I saw Ming come away from her supper, having left a little meat in the bowl as usual, and then I saw Emma, full of stealth, do a slow-motion walk towards the bowl. She was just about to put her great brown nose into it, when I shouted at her, 'Emma, leave it!'

It was as if someone had fired a shotgun behind her. She spun round, and looked at me with an expression I had never seen before: amazement, shock perhaps, even a hint that she had encountered the supernatural.

'Yes,' I said, 'I can see. You were going to finish that off, weren't you?' She came over to me, and pushed her nose into my hand, and wagged her tail rather tentatively, as if she wished to say: 'Well, what's all this about? I don't understand this at all.'

But I think she did understand, and knew from then on that I could see. After that, when she went on the lead, she started to pull, to bark at other dogs, and stop and sniff at lamp posts: things that the correct, dignified, working Emma would never have dreamt of doing. But now she did not have to work, nor, because she was eleven, was there any question of her being anyone else's guide dog. She had earned her freedom. When off the lead, she is a joy to watch, running along with her nose to the ground, stopping to investigate every tree and blade of grass, her tail waving high in the air. There were aspects of Emma I had never known about. How, for instance, her ears seemed to jump up and down as she ran. I love her energy and zest for life, and she seems to share my joy in being able to see her.

There were other things that also became clear to me as time went on. One thing, though I have never yet seen, and that is a rainbow. Don once rushed in to me in a storm when the sun was shining, and said, 'Come on, Sheila, come and look.' He was so excited. But by the time I was outside the sky had changed; everything had faded but for a faint bar of violet over the ground where the rainbow had been. He was immensely disappointed, and so was I. I am still waiting to catch a rainbow.

And, rainbow apart, at last I have now seen what Christmas is really like. Previously I had always felt sad at Christmas and frustrated because I knew the town would be decorated, with lights and Christmas trees and an enormous illuminated picture of Santa Claus, which I used to miss seeing most of all. And in the shops there would be a host of things that my mother would describe, but which I could never enjoy through window shopping. I could put out a hand and touch them, of course, but it is not the same. However (Don used to think it strange), I had always put up decorations at home. I would have my own impressions, knowing precisely where everything was, so that I could imagine the scene. I used to sit down, loving the idea that the house was properly decorated, and that I had done it. All those years of decorating for myself, and going shopping without being able to see what presents I was buying, dropped away as if they had never been. Being able to see and enjoy Christmas to the full, more than anything else, summed up what sight meant to me.

I bought more decorations than I had ever done before, and added them to the ones I already had. I also bought an enormous Christmas tree, and I hung tinsel everywhere. Don came home with some fairy lights, and when we switched them on – blue, orange, green – it was like being six again, only better. And the pleasure I had from writing my own Christmas cards, and from being able to know as soon as I opened the envelope who had sent us cards, was indescribable. On Christmas Day itself it was pure joy to watch Don open each present. Whether it was a shirt, or aftershave, I had chosen it myself.

Now another year has gone by, a year in which I have gradually become more used to, more practised in, what I can do with vision. But I have not, to this day, lost my sense of wonder. When I hear people in the street complaining about the price of potatoes or coal going up again, I want to remind them just how lucky they are simply to be able to see the sky and the clouds.

But Don and I think ourselves particularly lucky. Last Christmas brought an addition to the family. On 21 December I had a baby daughter, Kerensa Emma Louise, who is now ten weeks old. (The middle name was chosen, of course, for a very good chocolate-brown reason.) We have been blessed with a very beautiful baby. Don and I have happiness beyond all our dreams, and but one prayer left to be answered: that Kerensa will be able to see.

Afterword

2011

EMMA DIED THIRTY years ago, at the ripe old age of seventeen. I still miss her. Where could I find another friend who would be happy to stay with me at all times, be pleased when I wanted to go out, wherever I wanted to go, whenever I wanted to go? Emma had the most wonderful attitude towards life, one I try to emulate, that whatever she did, she was happy. Get in a car and she'd sleep till we got there. Get out and she'd enjoy the park, or meeting people, or snoozing under a table while I gave a talk, and she never complained. Friends like that are very hard to come by. That's what Emma was to me and she was also a part of me. I remember, people would stop me in the street and say, 'What a lovely dog you have,' and, for a moment, I would think, 'Dog, I don't have a dog.' I never thought of Emma as a dog, she was a person. We had six legs and a chocolate bit down one side.

When the book was first published, the three of us – myself, Don and Emma – travelled the length and breadth of Britain, to every radio station, television station and newspaper office. I so enjoyed that and so did Emma. We both enjoyed meeting people and I loved talking about Emma. She didn't care who they were, whether they were famous or infamous, everybody was the same. Although she had retired, she still had that special something, that intelligence that you don't often find in a pet dog. We were doing a chat show one evening and at the end of the show, the cameraman came up to me and said, 'Your dog is amazing.'

'Yes, of course she is.' I had just spent twenty minutes extolling her virtues on prime time television.

'No, I don't mean that.' He told me that she was behind my chair out of his view, and he had waved and gesticulated to her where he wanted her to go. She immediately got up and took centre stage.

Everyone recognised Emma after she had appeared on television and they all stopped and wanted to talk to her. If ever I went out without her, nobody stopped me and wanted to talk to me. They didn't recognise me without Emma by my side. We visited schools and WIs to tell them about Emma, opened fetes and judged dog shows. What a wonderful time.

I never, ever get fed up of talking about Emma. She left me so much: a legacy of knowing how clever dogs could be and that we really owe them so much more respect. I think dogs are capable of learning anything that they physically can do, if only we have the ability to communicate what we want.

Dogs came after Emma – chocolate Labradors, black Labradors and one or two German shorthaired pointers. I found it very difficult to adapt to having a pet/owner relationship. I expected the dogs to do things, to learn very quickly and to be as clever as Emma, but I had to train them. They were just puppies; they needed educating and guidance, just like children. I started taking them to training classes, but I realised that the people there were quite brutal. They put chains round the dogs' necks and shouted at them and bullied them into doing things. That wasn't the way I wanted to do it, so I learned by training my own dogs and competing at obedience shows, sorting out all the problems that I came across. I started my own dog training classes and, after a while, specialised in problem dogs. It's so rewarding to be able to help people with their dogs. Often, they are near the point of putting the dog down, thinking the problem can't be solved. My favourite part of the training is puppy classes. Puppies are so clever and so willing to learn, it's easy to train them. It's the owners who need the training and guidance. Some owners have no idea how to treat a puppy. They think the louder they shout, the more the puppy will obey them, whereas it is the reverse.

I want to give so much back because I have had so much happiness from dogs in the past. I was so lucky to meet Emma and so lucky to meet Don and then I had exactly what I wanted, a baby girl, Kerensa. We knew we were taking a risk, with a 50/50 chance of my eye defect passing on. We were so relieved when we discovered that her sight was perfect. Kerensa, of course, is an adult now and working as a Forensic Psychologist for the Prison Service. Don and I are still working, Don in his foot clinic and I am still training the dogs. We only have two dogs now – an old black Labrador and a German shorthaired pointer who was rescued from the RSPCA – and a Siamese cat. We have lived with as many as seven dogs in the house and five Siamese cats. It's a lot quieter these days.

I was given a wonderful opportunity by a charity called Dog AID to help disabled people train their dogs. Dog AID doesn't provide trained dogs but they help disabled people who already have a pet dog to train them. I was meeting people who were confined to wheelchairs and who had other disabilities, such as cerebral palsy or MS. I had some ideas about training dogs to help, but I had to set to work with my own dogs to find the best and easiest methods. Meeting these people certainly opened my eyes – if you will forgive the pun – to their individual needs. Someone confined to a wheelchair is going to find it difficult to retrieve and take some things around the house.

I feel privileged that I was able to help other disabled people train their pets. It involved training dogs to fetch named articles, like door keys or the telephone; to put clothes in the washing machine; to indicate where things are on the floor; and to generally assist their owners depending on their disability. For instance, I learned so much when training Cavendish, a Leonberger owned by Nicola, who desperately needed help with him, as she suffers from cerebral palsy and is visually impaired. Nicola and Cav had originally been taken on by another school training dogs for the disabled but he had been rejected on the grounds that he was aggressive. What had actually happened was, on one of his training sessions at the school, he had been attacked by a large dog and, from that point on, he became very stressed when dogs entered a room, or a training class situation. I realised it wasn't aggression, it was purely fear. I had to work out a very quick and easy way that Nicola could use to stop this happening and to reassure him, remembering that she wasn't going to get up and move quickly, and that she couldn't see whether people coming in the door had dogs or not. So we gave Cav something different to think about when a door opened and anyone entered: he would touch Nicola on the knee and she would reward him with a treat. This worked perfectly. It gave him something else to think about and he was rewarded every time someone with or without a dog entered the room. Nicola needed Cav to guide but for that he would have to be trained properly by the Guide Dogs for the Blind Association. However, they would only take him on if he had first been passed by one of the assistance dog organisations, so together we trained him up to pass. We taught him to fetch items, to assist Nicola when she needed physical help, and just to stand by her so she could put her hand on him for reassurance. Nicola had the added disability of not being able to walk properly and this can be very off-putting to a dog, so we had to get Cav used to being close to Nicola and allowing her to sometimes stop and rest. Nicola and Cav always gave me something new to think about and devise. Nicola told me they were going on a cruise. How would Cav adapt to a cabin situation? How could she train him very quickly to put important items in a place where she knew she could find them easily? Of course, he had a place at home to put things but we could hardly take the table and put it in a cabin on a cruise ship. I practiced various things with Bramble, a dog I had at the time who was incredibly intelligent. The answer was actually so simple. We used a bright yellow table mat, and wherever we put this table mat, the dog was trained to put the items we gave him. It worked like a charm. Nicola took the table mat into the cabin, put it down wherever she needed it and Cav would take the items she gave him and leave them on the mat.

We were all so pleased when Cav passed his test by Canine Partners to become a fully fledged dog for the disabled. He then went on to be trained by Guide Dogs and I believe he is one of the only dual-purpose dogs, certainly the only dual-purpose Leonberger, working in this country.

Dogs are like children, they love learning, especially if you make it fun – lots of rewards and no negative training. I soon learned that shouting at dogs or saying 'No' didn't work. We all want to be praised for the qualities that we have, not shouted at or grumbled at for the qualities that we don't have and things that we can't do. Animals are just the same so we should respect them. Emma taught me that. We enjoy being with people who are happy and don't moan, who are always pleased to see us. That's dogs for you.

I believe I have led a charmed life. Everything that has happened to me over the last 65 years has led to something good. I was so fortunate to have parents who were visually impaired, so I grew up as normal. I went to a normal school, I met Emma and Don, had Kerensa, and had some wonderful dogs over the years that have taught me so much. And now, I am doing exactly what I want to do to earn a living: training dogs.

Sheila Hocken